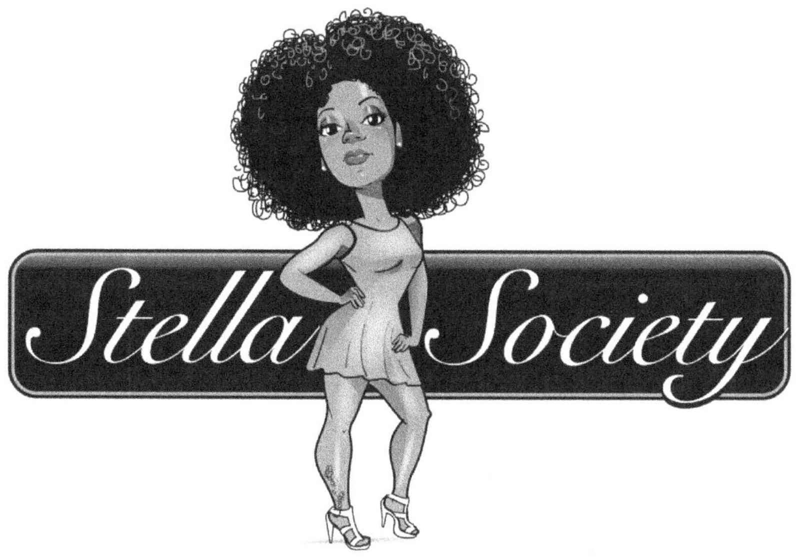

Thank you for participating in the Stella Project 2.0, a 40 day fitness confidence and nutrition challenge.
If you purchased this journal and you are not a member of the Stella Project, no worries. You can find us at stellasocietyacademy dot com, or just use it on your own 40 day fitness journey.

Always consult a physician before beginning an exercise program.

How to use your journal

Journaling has many benefits especially when tracking progress. Recording your thoughts before training can help you better understand why a workout did or didn't go too well. Recalling the times you eat and what can help you combat unnecessary cravings. Journaling also increases self-discipline, improves your mood and boost comprehension. Please use this journal to aid in your goals through your 40 days.

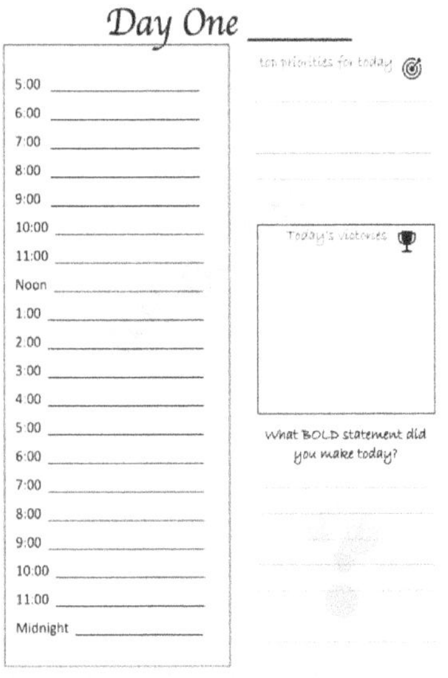

Use this page to record your daily schedule, meals, training, meetings, etc. Make sure you put the date. List your top priorities hat must be completed that day. Record your victories, like drinking all your water and reflect on the daily bestellatude

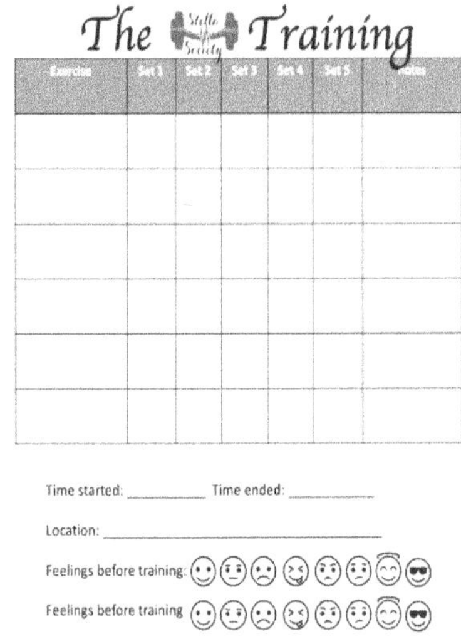

Use this page to record your training sessions. Write them down ahead of time and watch the video in case you have questions. Put the time your started and completed the training as well as how you felt before and after. Leave a note as to why you felt a certain before the training. This could effect how it went.

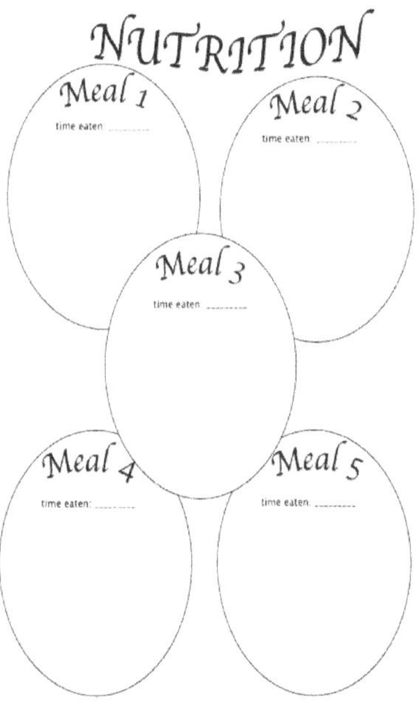

Use this page to record your meals and the time you ate them. This is important especially when tracking your progress. Try to eat your meals at the same time each day. Get your machine on a schedule so it knows how to operate its fuel.

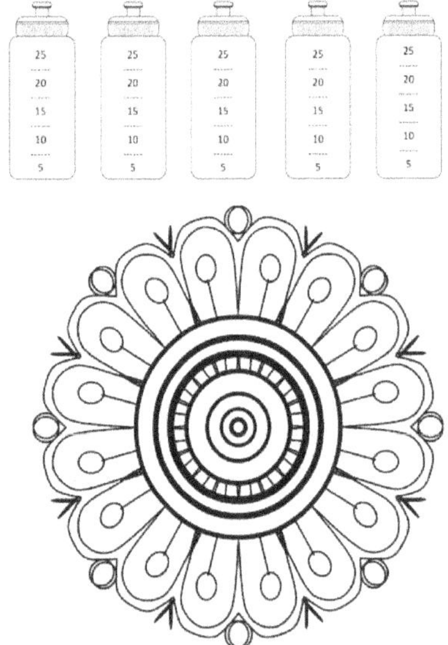

Use this page to record your water intake. Color the bottles as you complete each one. Also each hydration page has a mandala graphic to color. Coloring is a form of meditation. Choose to color this instead of reaching for something to snack on that's not you're your meal plan.

R.O.S.E.S GOAL

Rationale – why are you participating in this 40 day challenge?

____

____

Objective – what do you look to accomplish during the 40 days? What is the end game, goal?

____

____

Strategy – how will you go about completing your objective? What actions will you take.

____

____

Evaluation – how and when will you evaluate you progress? Will you use inches, weight, look, or clothes?

____

____

Schedule – create a schedule for the next 40 days. Include anything that will get in the way of your goal and find a work around.

____

____

Measurements

DATE: __________

Weight: _______

Neck _______

Shoulders _______

Chest _______

Bicep / upper arm left _________ right _______

Forearm left _______ right _______

Waist _______

Hips _______

Thighs left _________ right _______

Calf left _______ right _______

Only I Can Change My Life, No One Can Do It For Me

Day One _______

____
____
____
____
____

5:00 ____________________
6:00 ____________________
7:00 ____________________
8:00 ____________________
9:00 ____________________
10:00 ____________________
11:00 ____________________
Noon ____________________
1:00 ____________________
2:00 ____________________
3:00 ____________________
4:00 ____________________
5:00 ____________________
6:00 ____________________
7:00 ____________________
8:00 ____________________
9:00 ____________________
10:00 ____________________
11:00 ____________________
Midnight ____________________

Today's victories

What BOLD statement did you make today?

____
____
____
____
____
____

The Training

Exercise	Set 1	Set 2	Set 3	Set 4	Set 5	notes

Time started: _____________   Time ended: _______________

Location: ____

Feelings before training:

Feelings after training

NUTRITION

Meal 1
time eaten: _________

Meal 2
time eaten: _________

Meal 3
time eaten: _________

Meal 4
time eaten: _________

Meal 5
time eaten: _________

Hydration

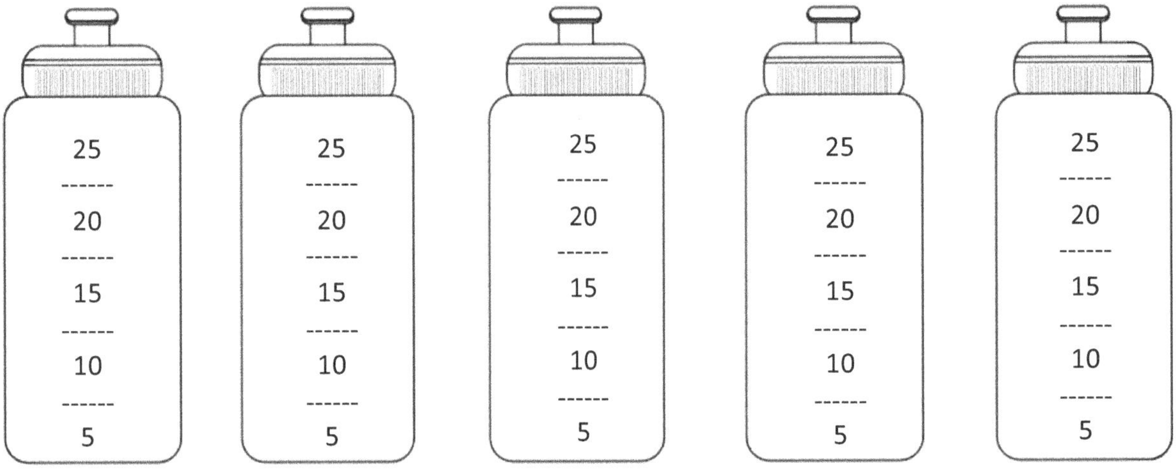

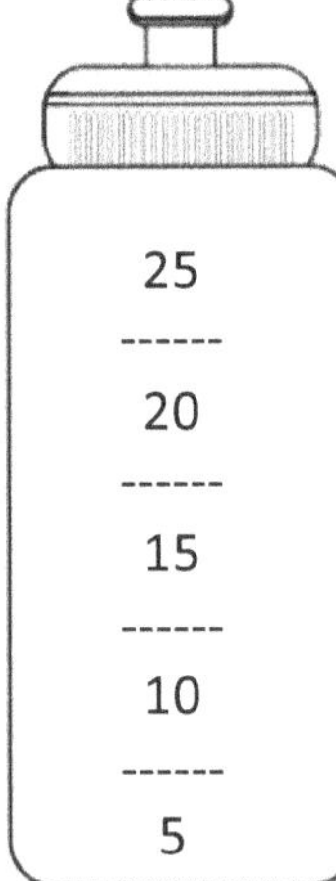

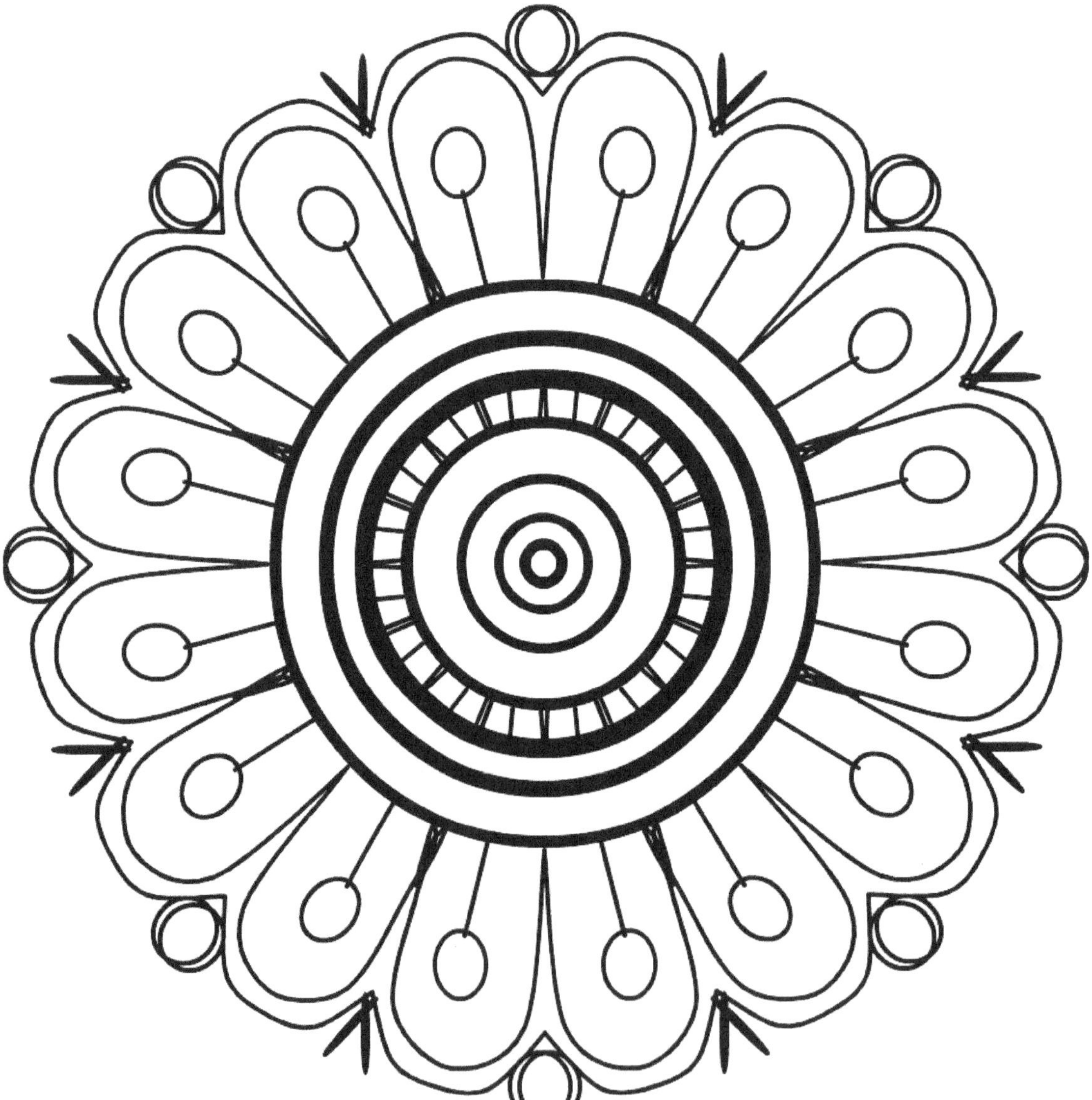

Day Two _______

5:00 ______________________	

5:00 ___________________

6:00 ___________________

7:00 ___________________

8:00 ___________________

9:00 ___________________

10:00 ___________________

11:00 ___________________

Noon ___________________

1:00 ___________________

2:00 ___________________

3:00 ___________________

4:00 ___________________

5:00 ___________________

6:00 ___________________

7:00 ___________________

8:00 ___________________

9:00 ___________________

10:00 ___________________

11:00 ___________________

Midnight ___________________

top priorities for today

____

____

____

____

Today's victories

What is one thing that makes you unique??

____

____

____

____

____

____

The Training

Exercise	Set 1	Set 2	Set 3	Set 4	Set 5	notes

Time started: _____________ Time ended: _______________

Location: ____

Feelings before training:

Feelings after training

NUTRITION

Meal 1

time eaten: _________

Meal 2

time eaten: _________

Meal 3

time eaten: _________

Meal 4

time eaten: _________

Meal 5

time eaten: _________

Hydration

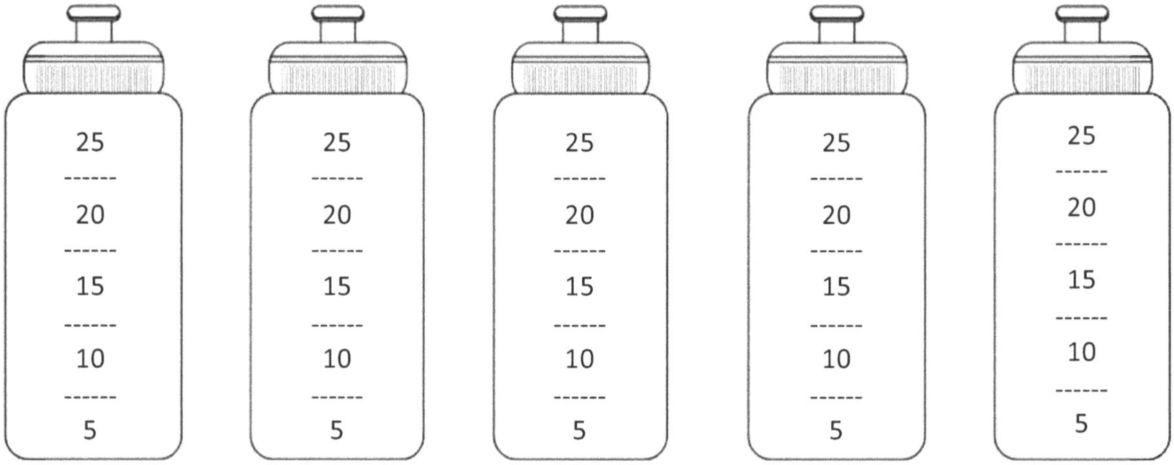

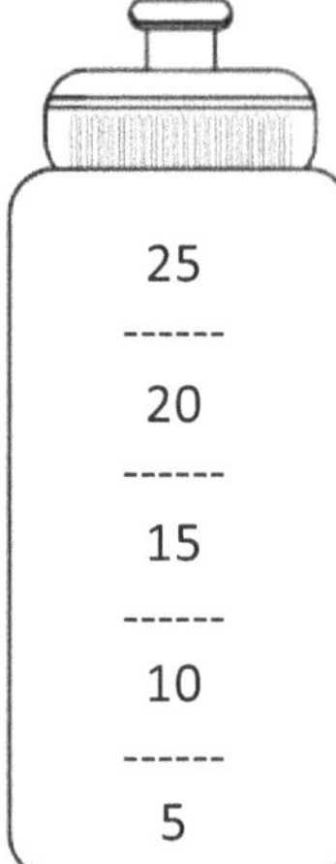 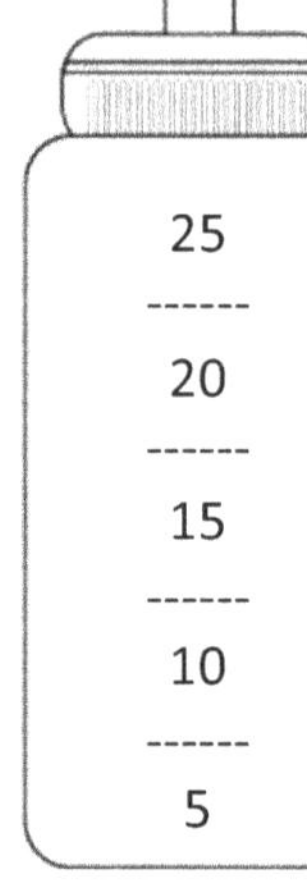 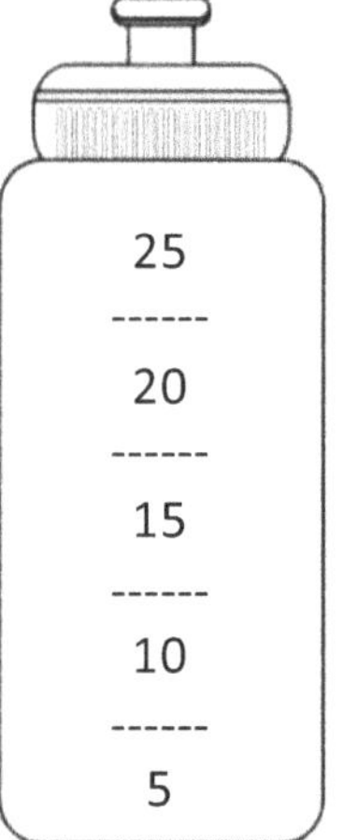

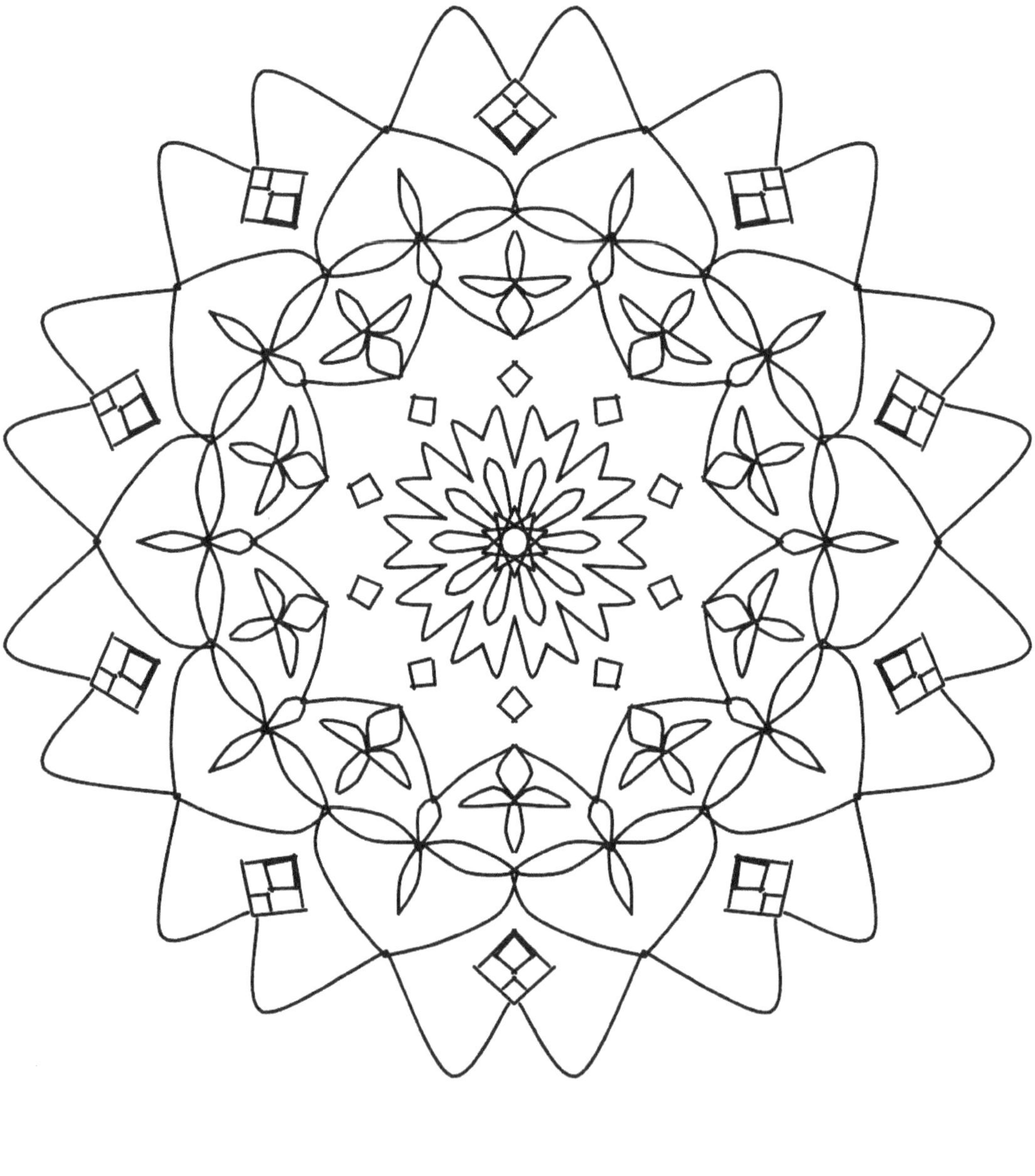

Day Three __________

5:00 _________________________

6:00 _________________________

7:00 _________________________

8:00 _________________________

9:00 _________________________

10:00 _________________________

11:00 _________________________

Noon _________________________

1:00 _________________________

2:00 _________________________

3:00 _________________________

4:00 _________________________

5:00 _________________________

6:00 _________________________

7:00 _________________________

8:00 _________________________

9:00 _________________________

10:00 _________________________

11:00 _________________________

Midnight _________________________

top priorities for today

Today's victories

What makes you brave?

The Training

Exercise	Set 1	Set 2	Set 3	Set 4	Set 5	notes

Time started: _____________ Time ended: _______________

Location: ____

Feelings before training:

Feelings after training

NUTRITION

Meal 1
time eaten: _________

Meal 2
time eaten: _________

Meal 3
time eaten: _________

Meal 4
time eaten: _________

Meal 5
time eaten: _________

Hydration

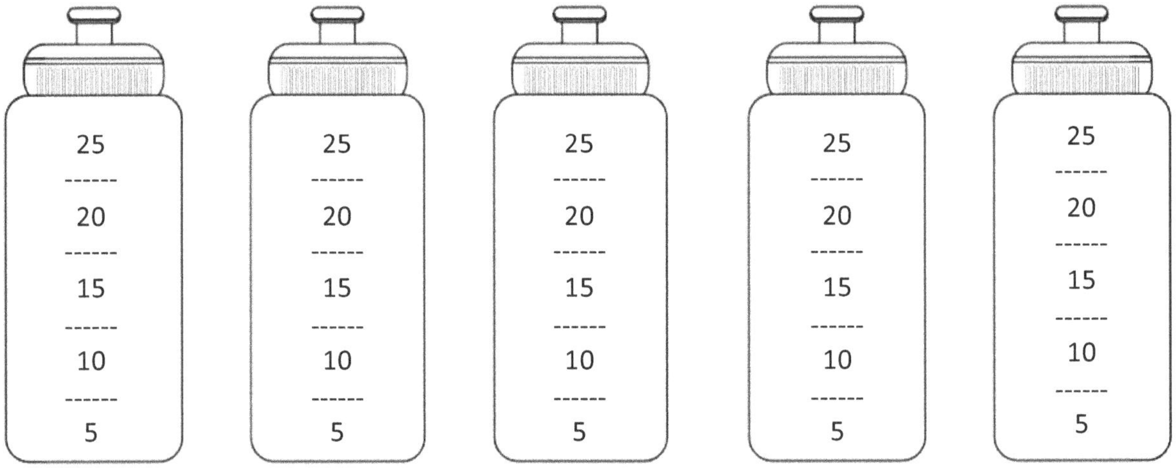

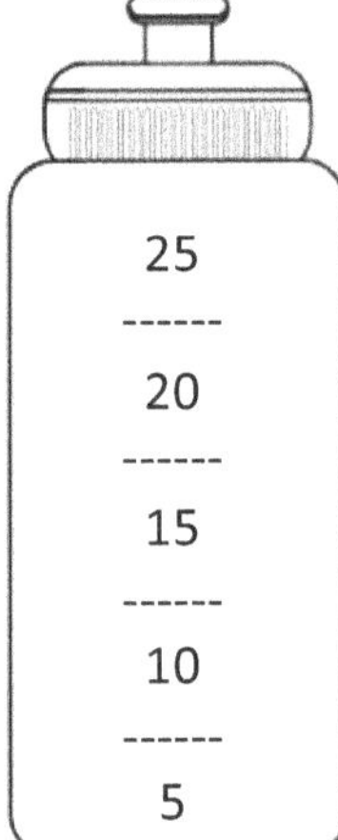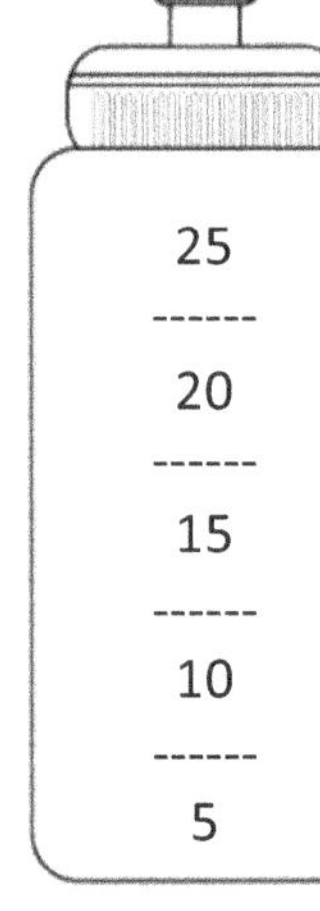

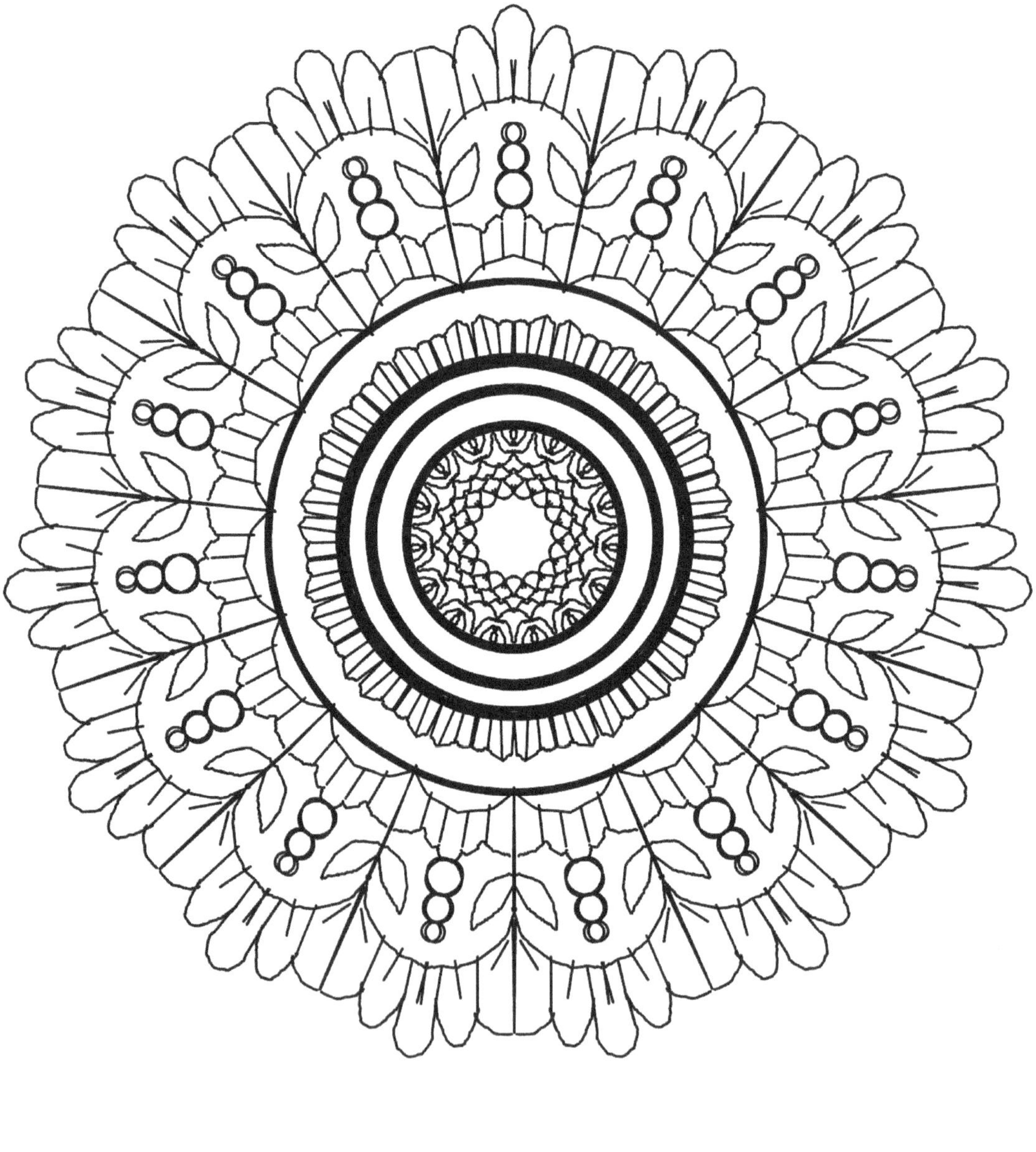

Day Four _______

5:00 _______________________

6:00 _______________________

7:00 _______________________

8:00 _______________________

9:00 _______________________

10:00 ______________________

11:00 ______________________

Noon _______________________

1:00 _______________________

2:00 _______________________

3:00 _______________________

4:00 _______________________

5:00 _______________________

6:00 _______________________

7:00 _______________________

8:00 _______________________

9:00 _______________________

10:00 ______________________

11:00 ______________________

Midnight ___________________

top priorities for today

____

____

____

____

Today's victories

What did you commit to today that will make for a better tomorrow?

____

____

____

____

____

____

____

The Stella Society Training

Exercise	Set 1	Set 2	Set 3	Set 4	Set 5	notes

Time started: _____________ Time ended: _______________

Location: ____

Feelings before training:

Feelings aftertraining

NUTRITION

Meal 1

time eaten: _________

Meal 2

time eaten: _________

Meal 3

time eaten: _________

Meal 4

time eaten: _________

Meal 5

time eaten: _________

Hydration

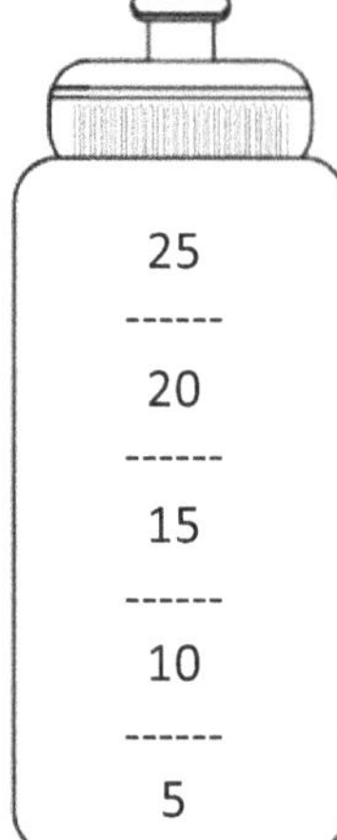

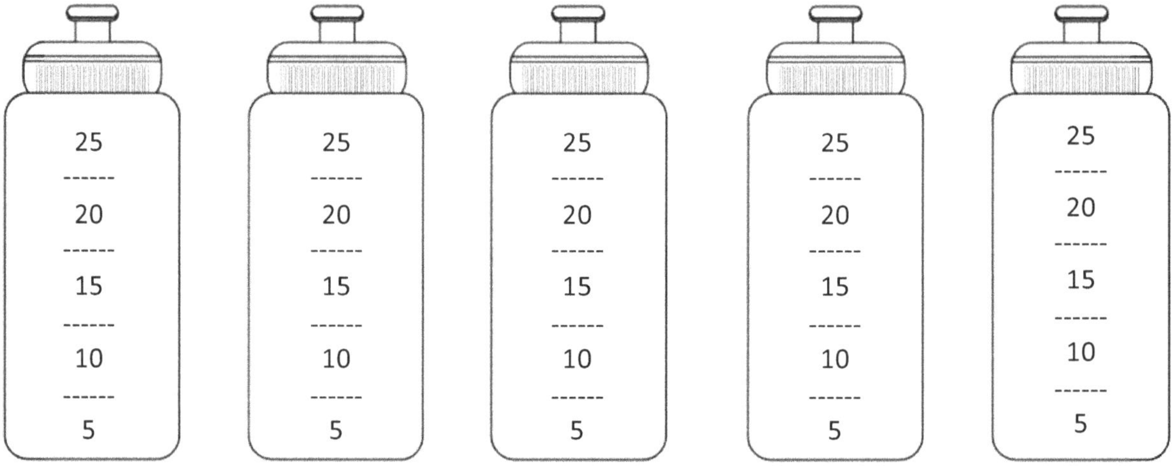

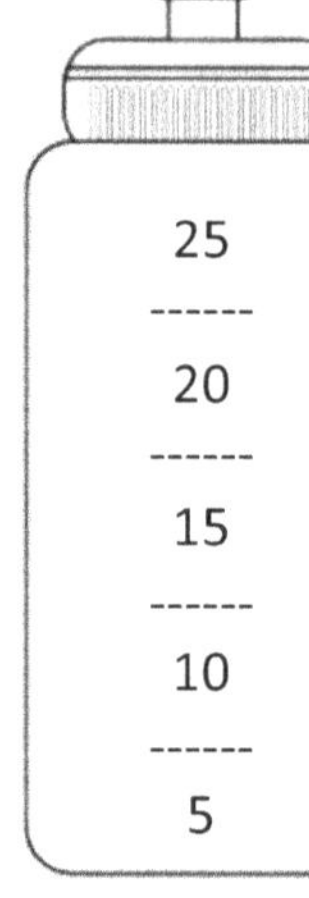

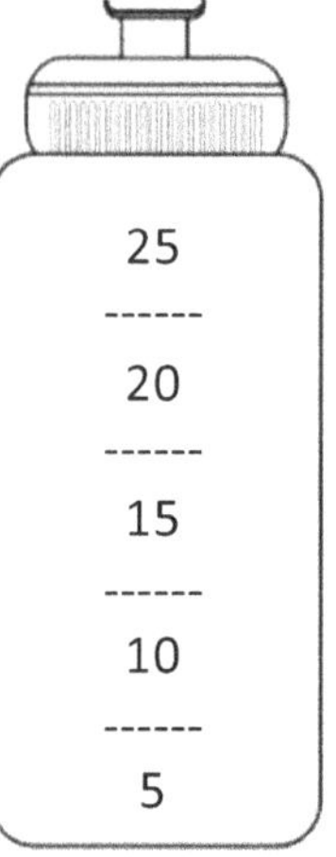

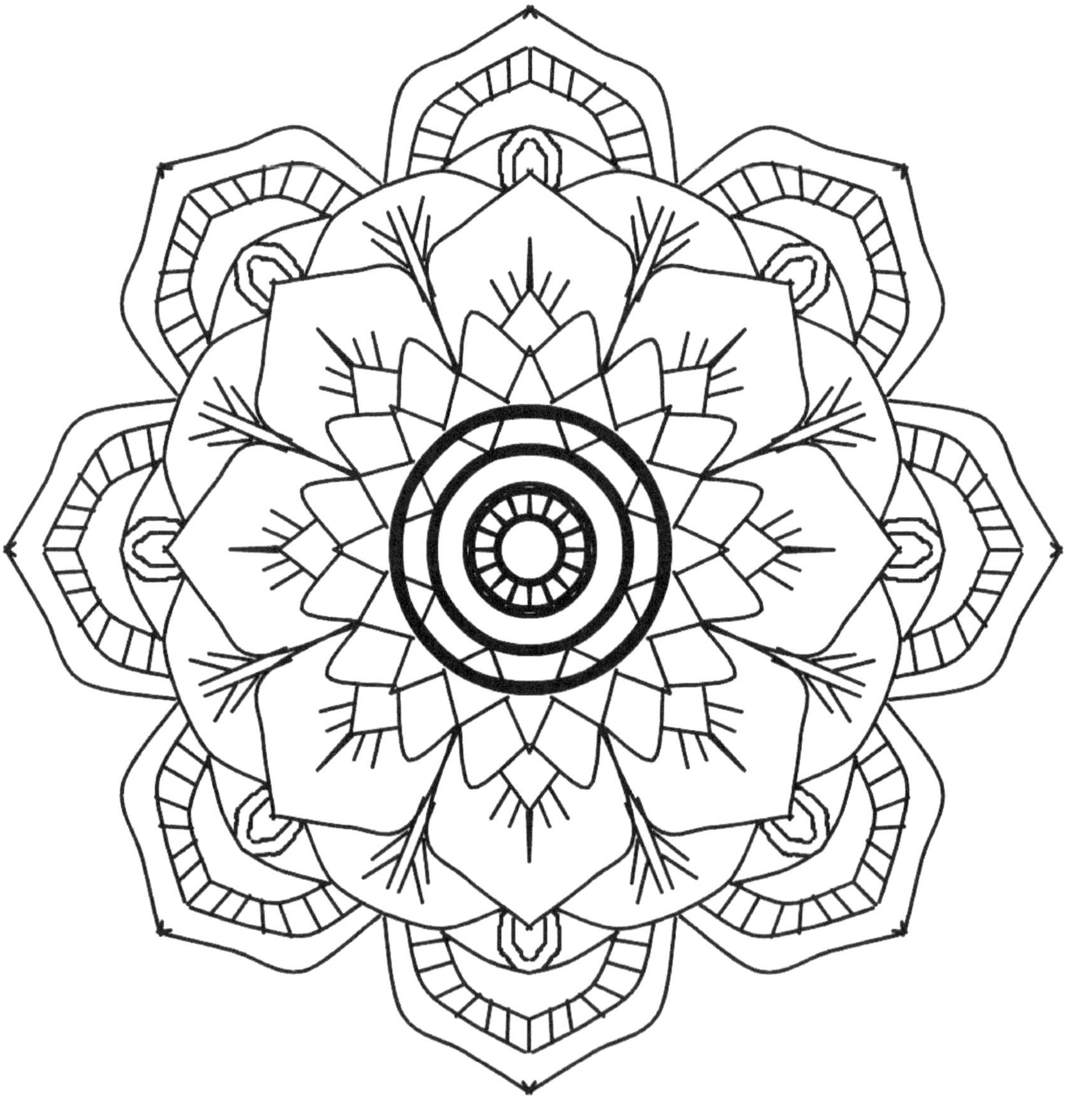

Day Five ______

5:00 ____________________	

5:00 ____________________

6:00 ____________________

7:00 ____________________

8:00 ____________________

9:00 ____________________

10:00 ____________________

11:00 ____________________

Noon ____________________

1:00 ____________________

2:00 ____________________

3:00 ____________________

4:00 ____________________

5:00 ____________________

6:00 ____________________

7:00 ____________________

8:00 ____________________

9:00 ____________________

10:00 ____________________

11:00 ____________________

Midnight ____________________

top priorities for today 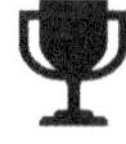

____

____

____

____

Today's victories

Who is the wisest person you know?
Talk to them today.

____

____

____

____

____

____

The Training

Exercise	Set 1	Set 2	Set 3	Set 4	Set 5	notes

Time started: _____________ Time ended: ______________

Location: ____

Feelings before training:

Feelings after training

NUTRITION

Meal 1

time eaten: _________

Meal 2

time eaten: _________

Meal 3

time eaten: _________

Meal 4

time eaten: _________

Meal 5

time eaten: _________

Hydration

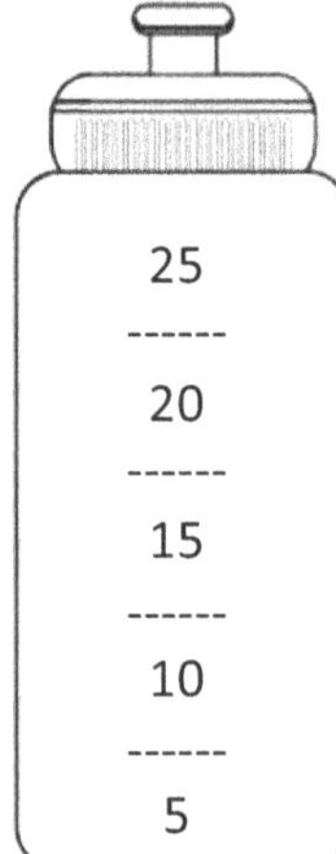
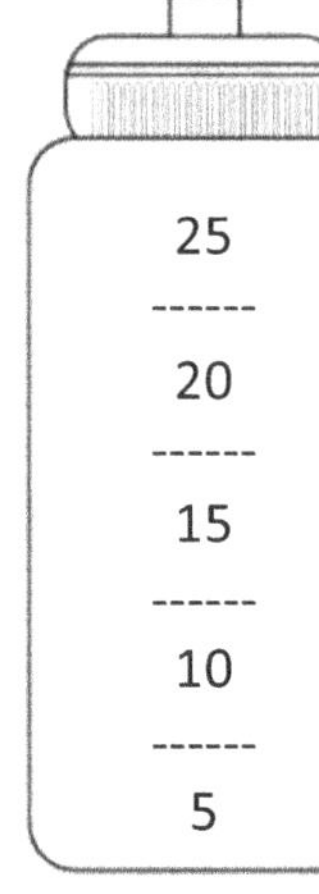

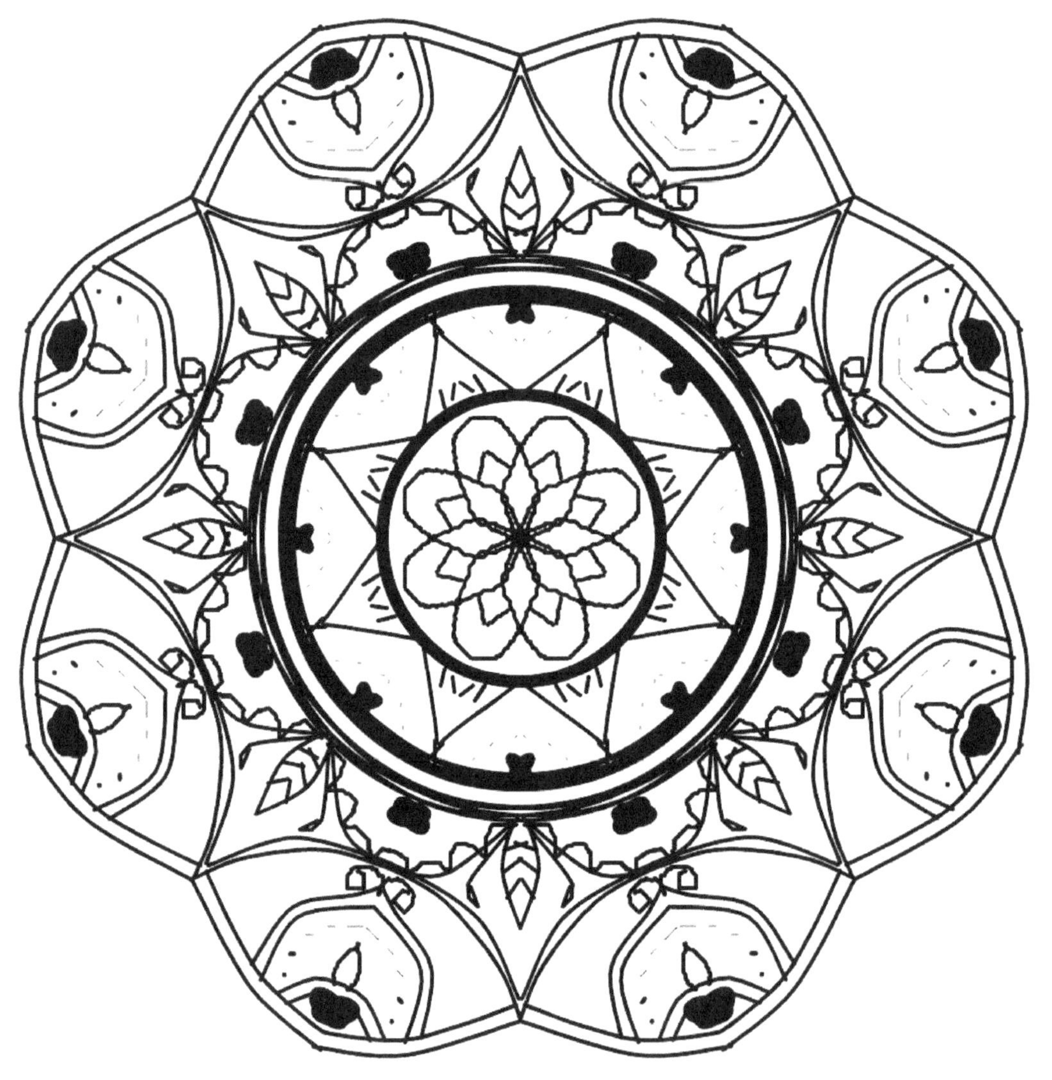

Day Six _______

5:00 _______________________

6:00 _______________________

7:00 _______________________

8:00 _______________________

9:00 _______________________

10:00 _______________________

11:00 _______________________

Noon _______________________

1:00 _______________________

2:00 _______________________

3:00 _______________________

4:00 _______________________

5:00 _______________________

6:00 _______________________

7:00 _______________________

8:00 _______________________

9:00 _______________________

10:00 _______________________

11:00 _______________________

Midnight _______________________

top priorities for today

____

____

____

____

____

Today's victories

What is your biggest fear and how do you get over it?

____

____

____

____

____

____

The Training

Exercise	Set 1	Set 2	Set 3	Set 4	Set 5	notes

Time started: _____________ Time ended: _______________

Location: ____

Feelings before training:

Feelings after training

NUTRITION

Meal 1

time eaten: _________

Meal 2

time eaten: _________

Meal 3

time eaten: _________

Meal 4

time eaten: _________

Meal 5

time eaten: _________

Hydration

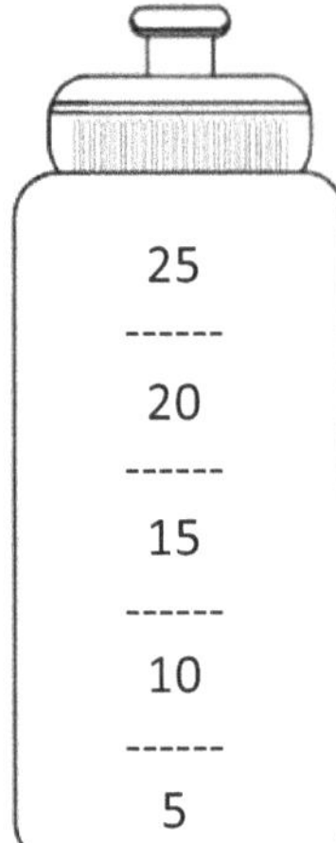
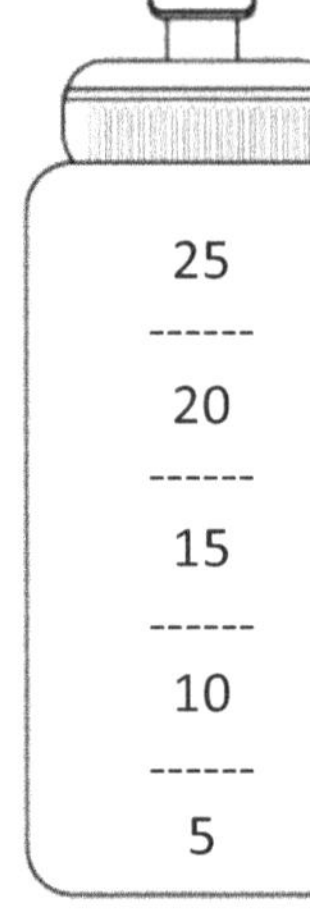
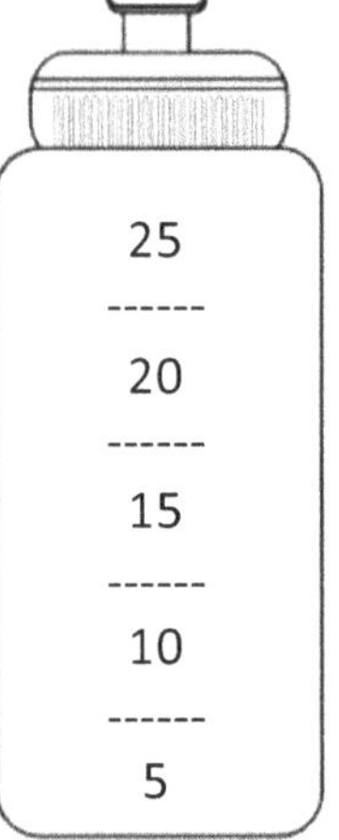
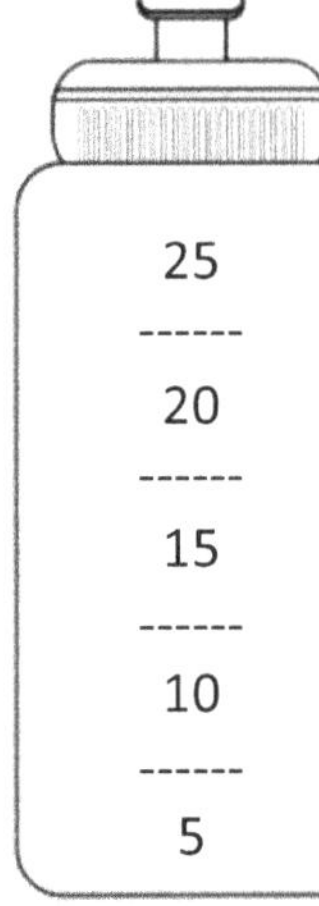
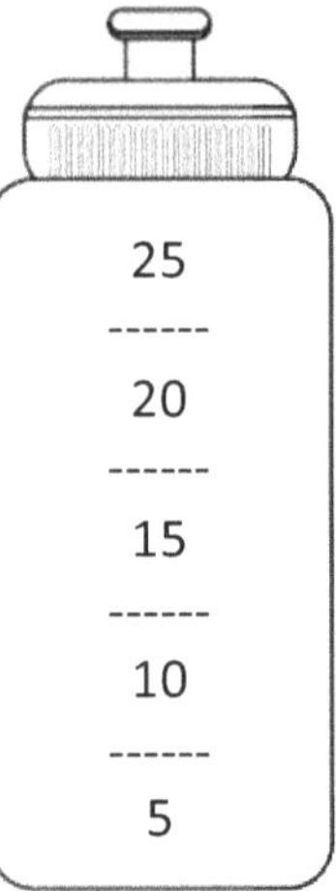

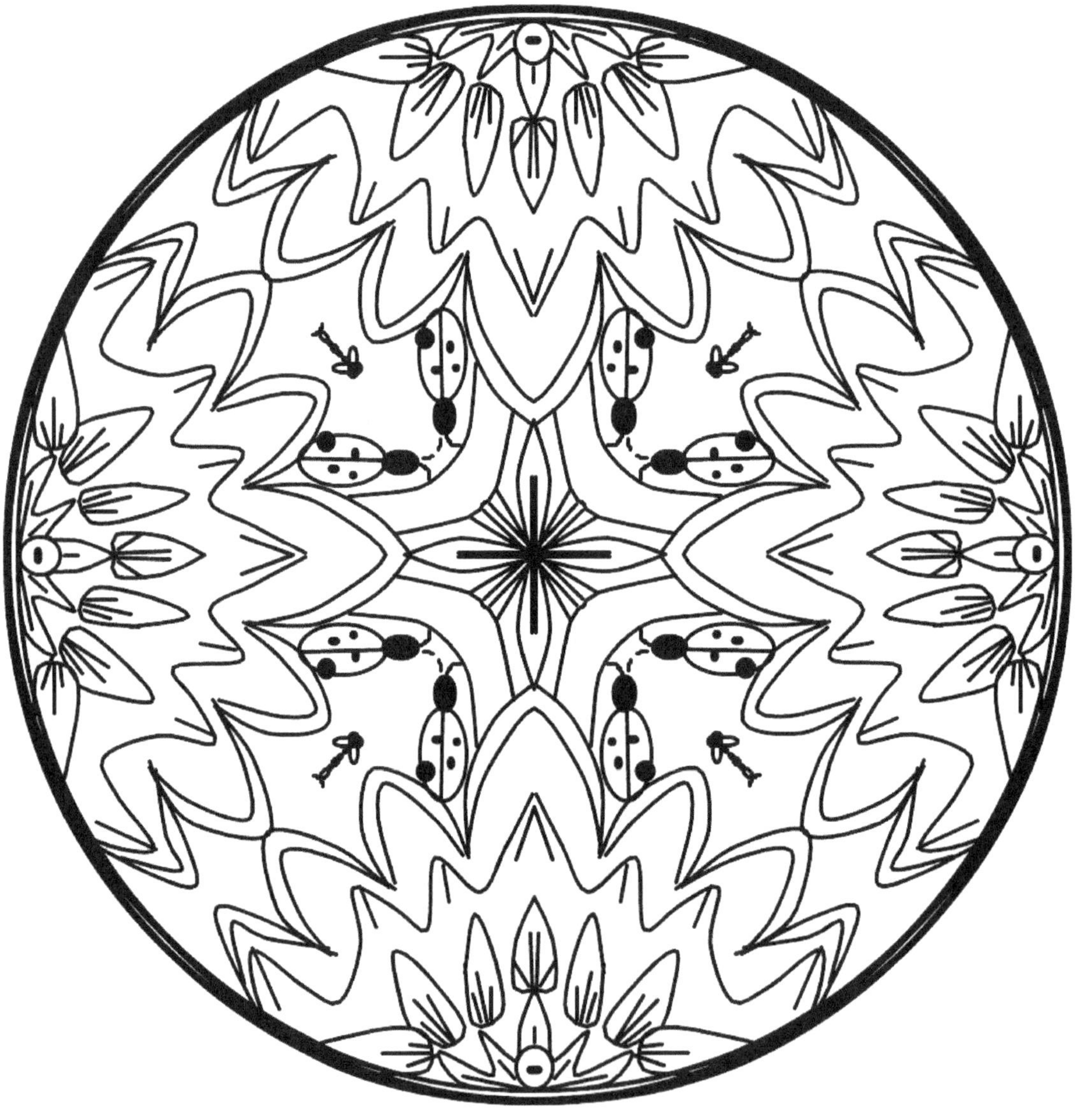

Day Seven _______

5:00 _____________________	

5:00 _______________________

6:00 _______________________

7:00 _______________________

8:00 _______________________

9:00 _______________________

10:00 ______________________

11:00 ______________________

Noon ______________________

1:00 _______________________

2:00 _______________________

3:00 _______________________

4:00 _______________________

5:00 _______________________

6:00 _______________________

7:00 _______________________

8:00 _______________________

9:00 _______________________

10:00 ______________________

11:00 ______________________

Midnight ___________________

top priorities for today

____

____

____

____

Today's victories

Where does your strength
come from?

____

____

____

____

____

____

____

The Stella Society Training

Exercise	Set 1	Set 2	Set 3	Set 4	Set 5	notes

Time started: _____________ Time ended: _______________

Location: ____

Feelings before training:

Feelings after training

NUTRITION

Meal 1
time eaten: _________

Meal 2
time eaten: _________

Meal 3
time eaten: _________

Meal 4
time eaten: _________

Meal 5
time eaten: _________

Hydration

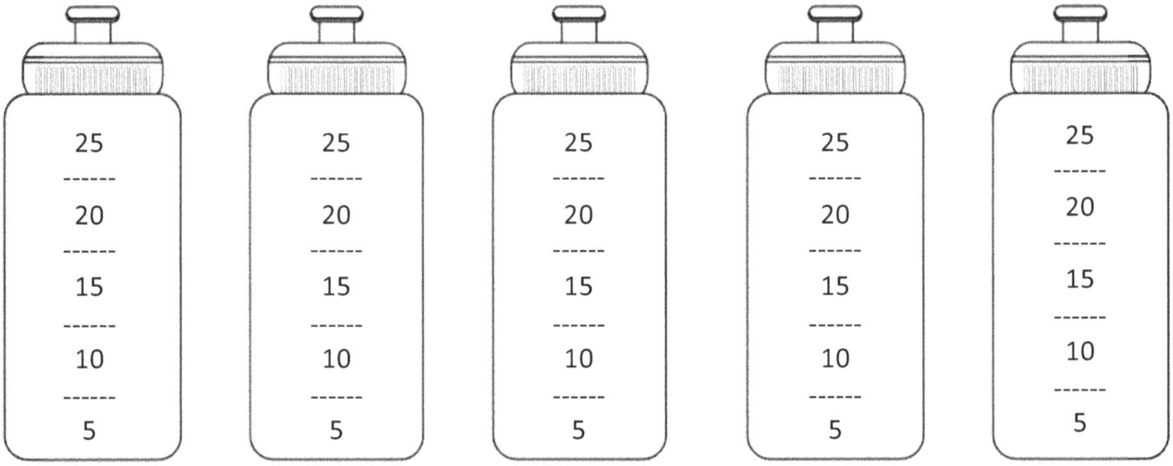

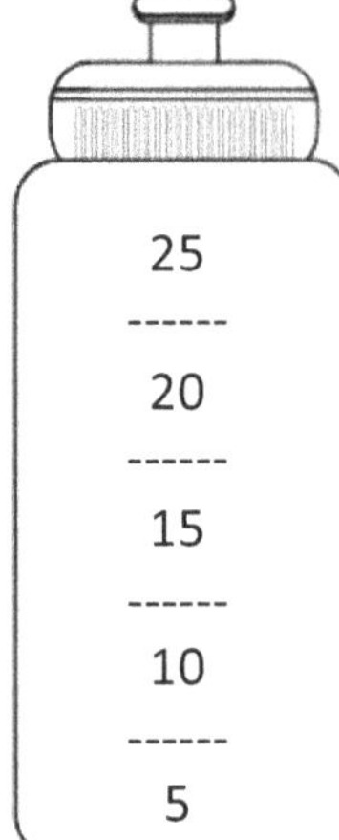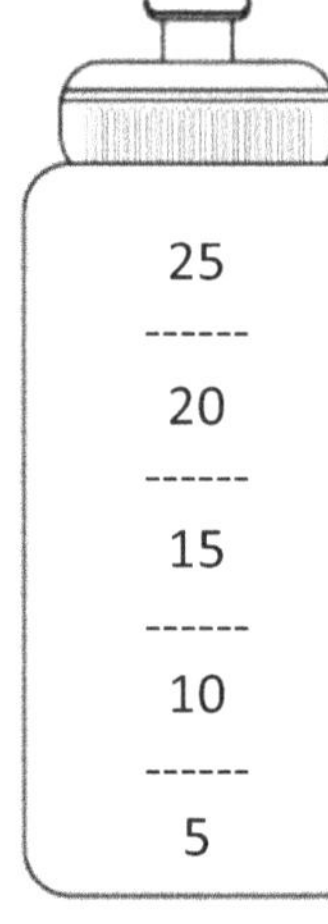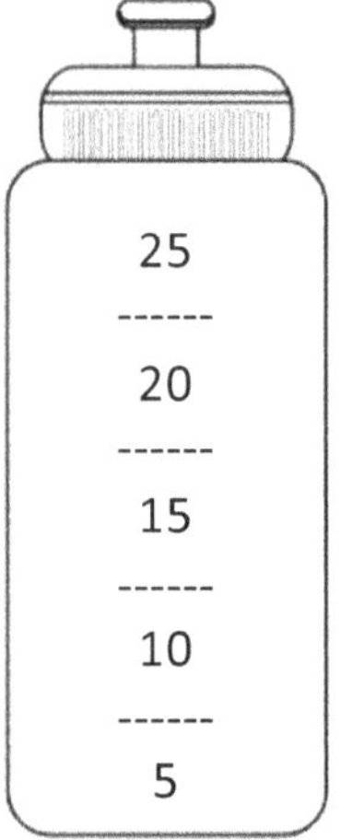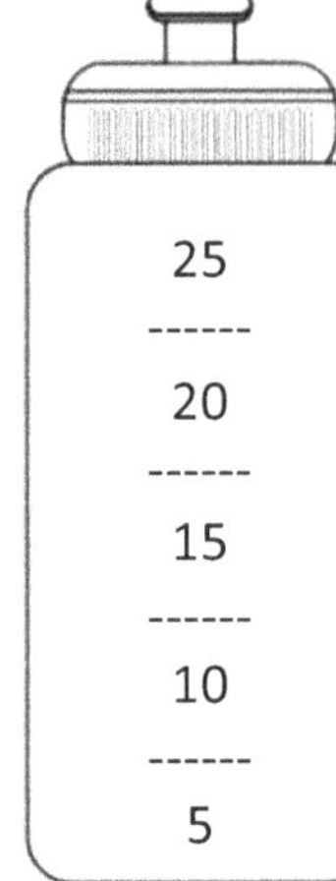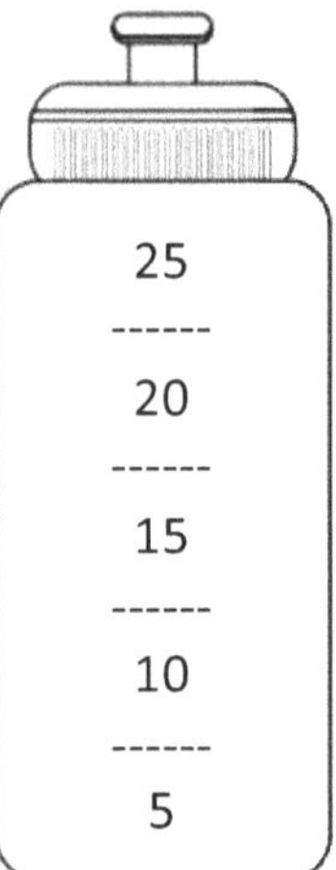

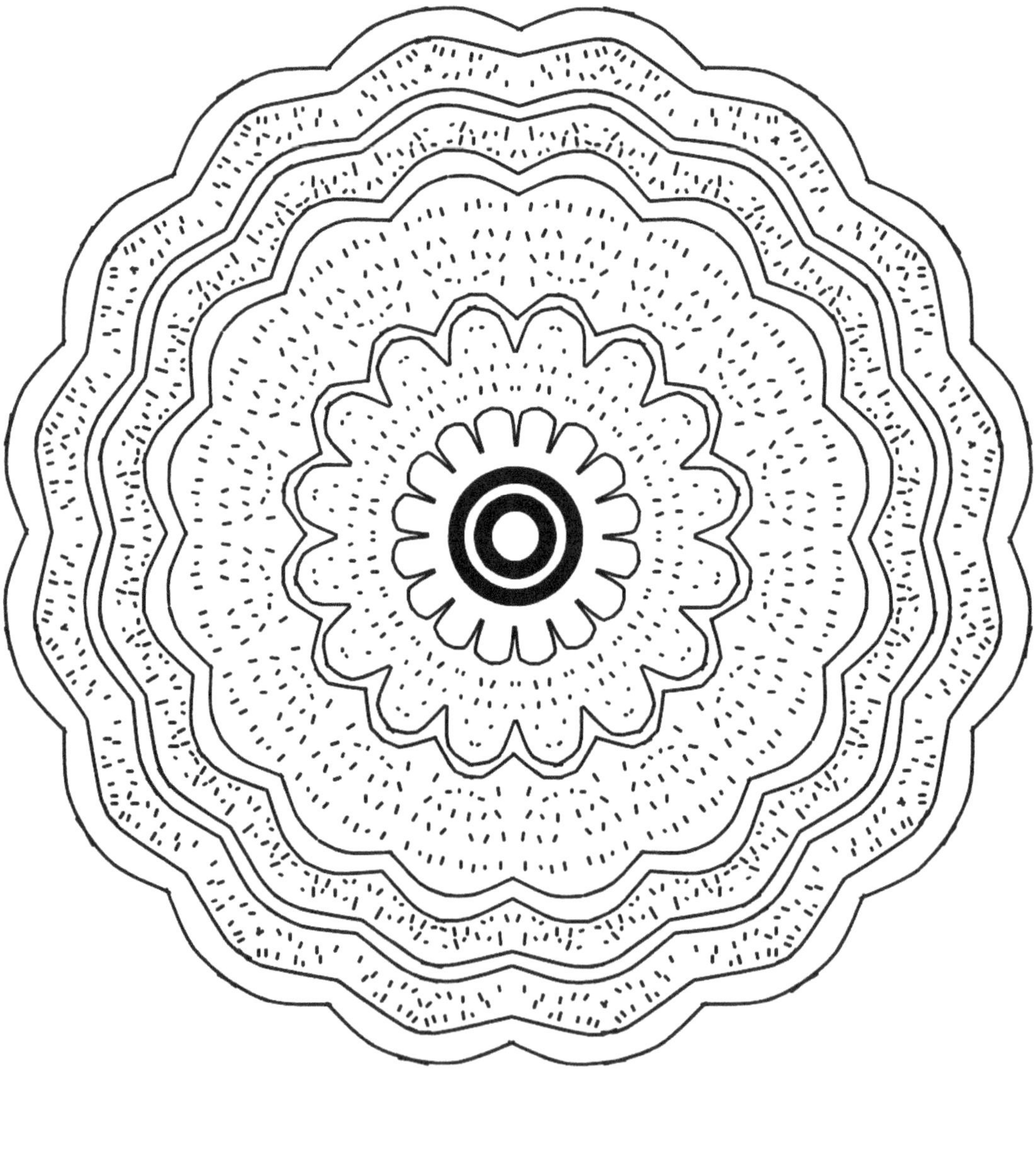

Day Eight ______

5:00 __________________	

5:00 ________________________

6:00 ________________________

7:00 ________________________

8:00 ________________________

9:00 ________________________

10:00 ______________________

11:00 ______________________

Noon ______________________

1:00 ________________________

2:00 ________________________

3:00 ________________________

4:00 ________________________

5:00 ________________________

6:00 ________________________

7:00 ________________________

8:00 ________________________

9:00 ________________________

10:00 ______________________

11:00 ______________________

Midnight __________________

What motivates you to be
the best version of you?

The Training

Exercise	Set 1	Set 2	Set 3	Set 4	Set 5	notes

Time started: _____________ Time ended: _______________

Location: ____

Feelings before training:

Feelings after training

NUTRITION

Meal 1
time eaten: _________

Meal 2
time eaten: _________

Meal 3
time eaten: _________

Meal 4
time eaten: _________

Meal 5
time eaten: _________

Hydration

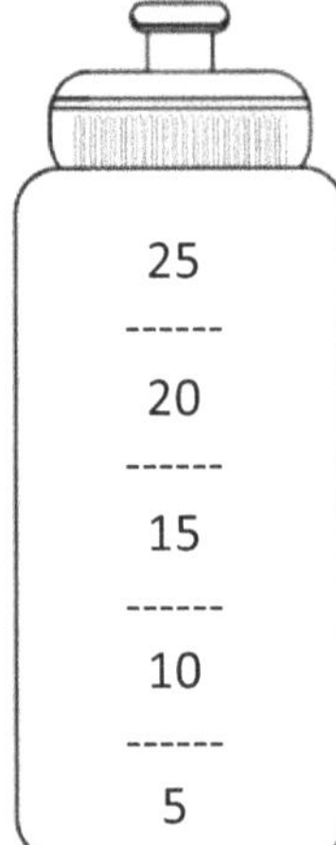

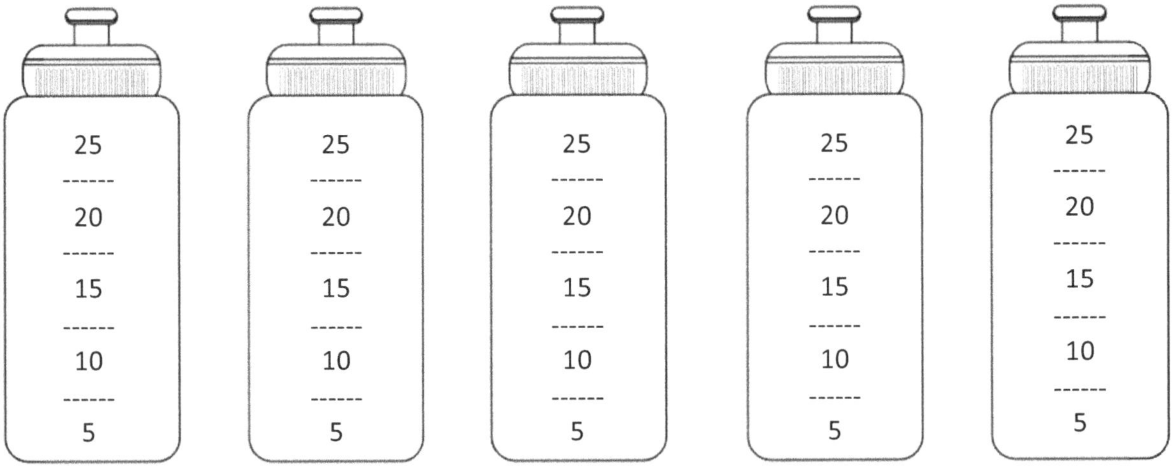

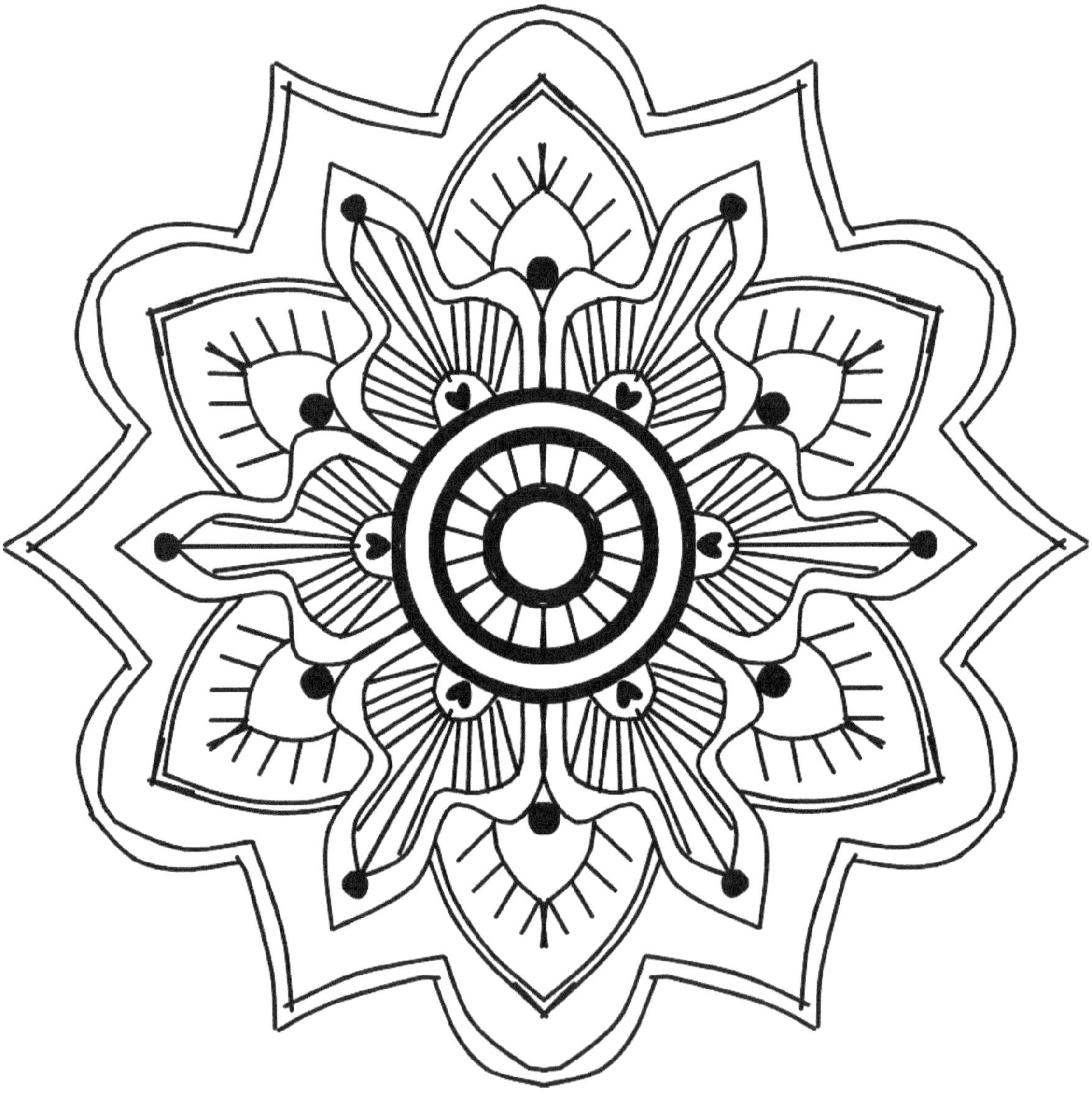

Day Nine _______

5:00 _______________________

6:00 _______________________

7:00 _______________________

8:00 _______________________

9:00 _______________________

10:00 _______________________

11:00 _______________________

Noon _______________________

1:00 _______________________

2:00 _______________________

3:00 _______________________

4:00 _______________________

5:00 _______________________

6:00 _______________________

7:00 _______________________

8:00 _______________________

9:00 _______________________

10:00 _______________________

11:00 _______________________

Midnight _______________________

top priorities for today

____

____

____

____

Today's victories

How will you be consistent this week?

____

____

____

____

____

____

The Stella Society Training

Exercise	Set 1	Set 2	Set 3	Set 4	Set 5	notes

Time started: _____________   Time ended: ______________

Location: ____

Feelings before training: 🙂 😐 🙁 😜 😣 😟 😇 😎

Feelings after training 🙂 😐 🙁 😜 😣 😟 😇 😎

NUTRITION

Meal 1

time eaten: _________

Meal 2

time eaten: _________

Meal 3

time eaten: _________

Meal 4

time eaten: _________

Meal 5

time eaten: _________

Hydration

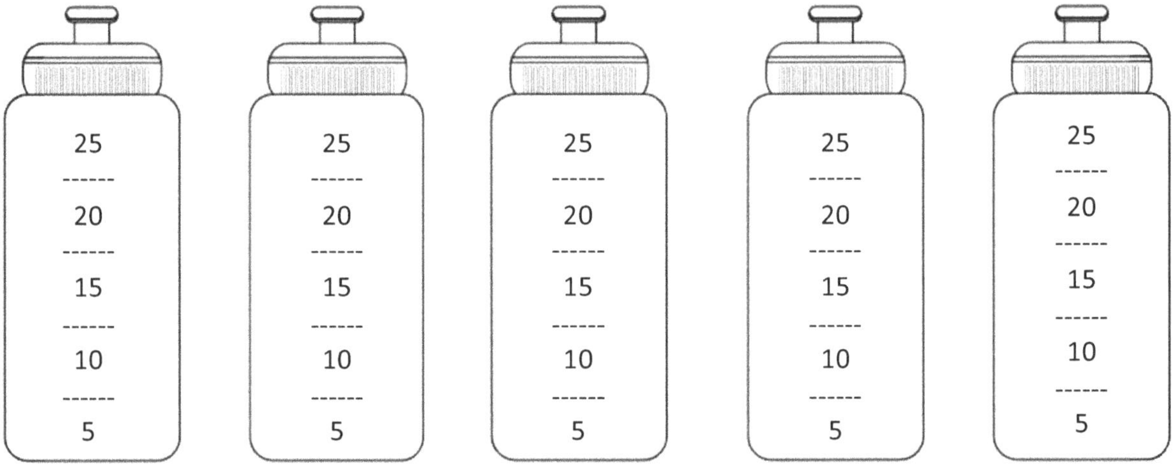

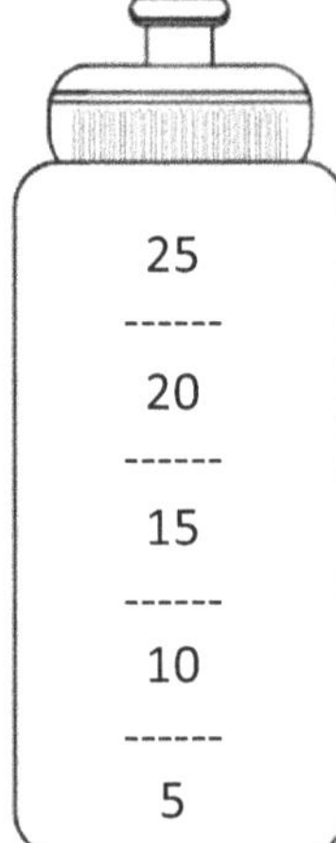
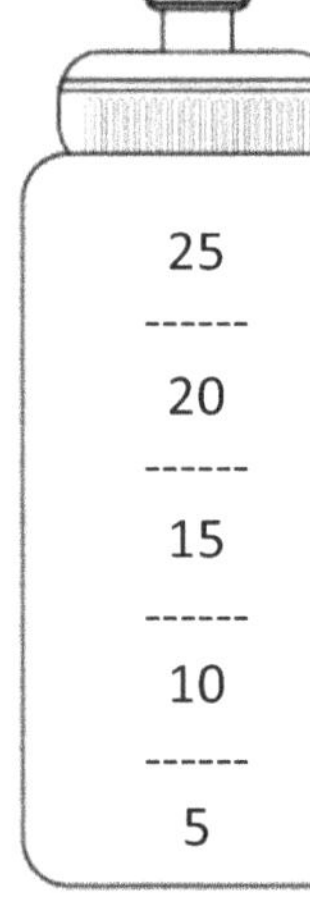

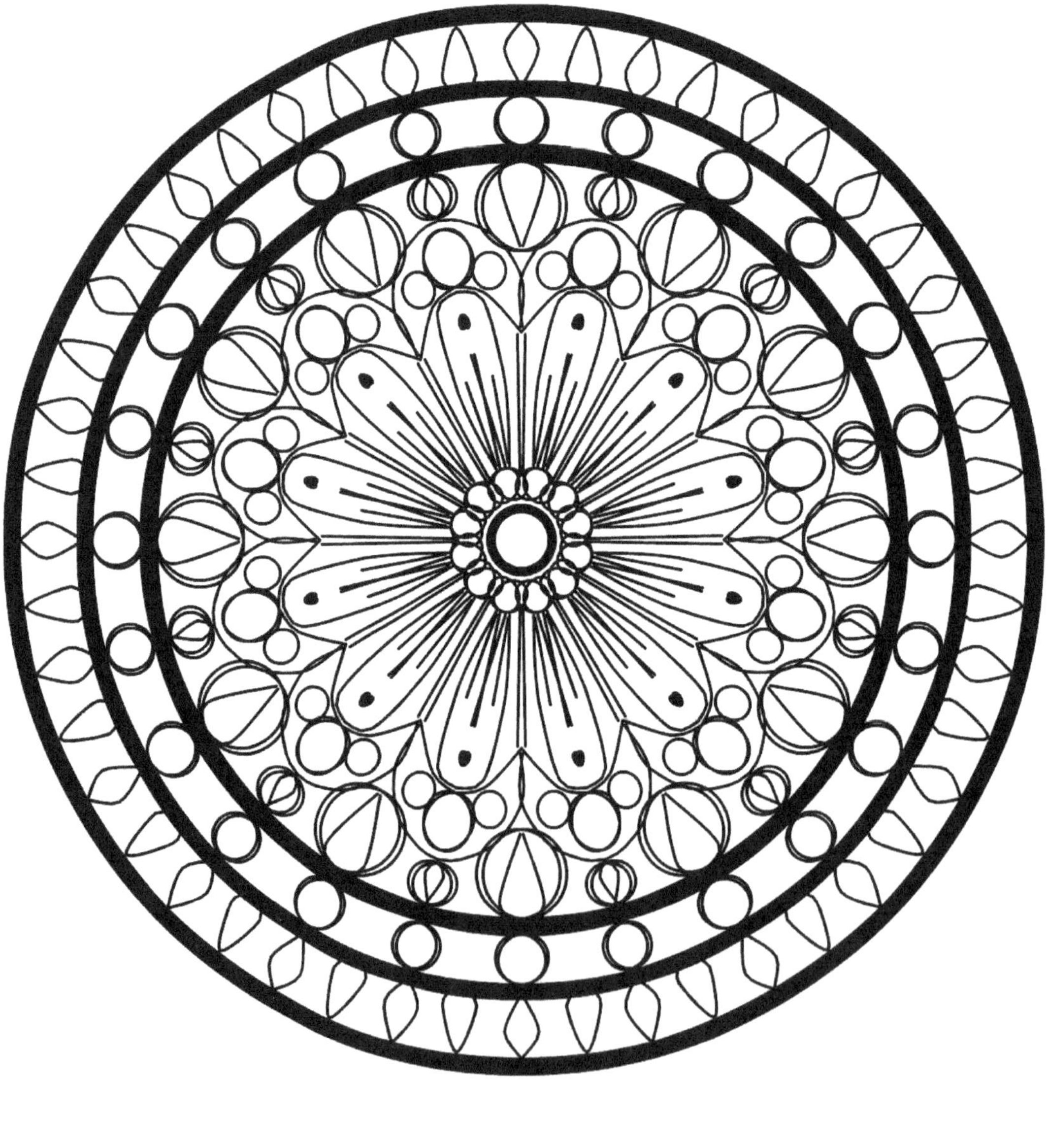

Day Ten _______

5:00 _____________________________

6:00 _____________________________

7:00 _____________________________

8:00 _____________________________

9:00 _____________________________

10:00 _____________________________

11:00 _____________________________

Noon _____________________________

1:00 _____________________________

2:00 _____________________________

3:00 _____________________________

4:00 _____________________________

5:00 _____________________________

6:00 _____________________________

7:00 _____________________________

8:00 _____________________________

9:00 _____________________________

10:00 _____________________________

11:00 _____________________________

Midnight _____________________________

top priorities for today

____

____

____

____

Today's victories

List 5 ways you are loving.

____

____

____

____

____

____

____

The *Stella Society* Training

Exercise	Set 1	Set 2	Set 3	Set 4	Set 5	notes

Time started: _____________ Time ended: _____________

Location: ____

Feelings before training: 🙂 😐 🙁 😜 😠 😟 😊 😎

Feelings after training 🙂 😐 🙁 😜 😠 😟 😊 😎

NUTRITION

Meal 1

time eaten: _________

Meal 2

time eaten: _________

Meal 3

time eaten: _________

Meal 4

time eaten: _________

Meal 5

time eaten: _________

Hydration

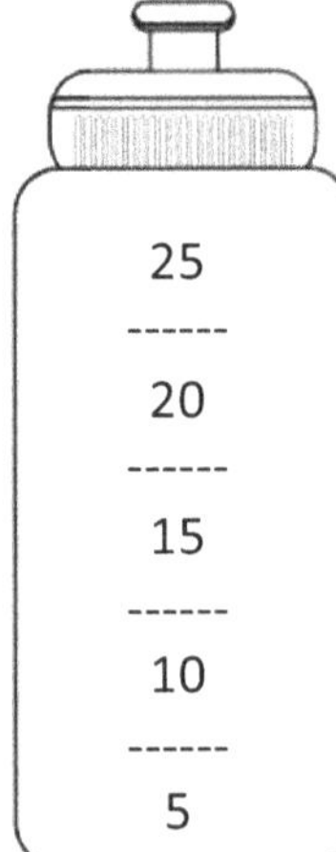

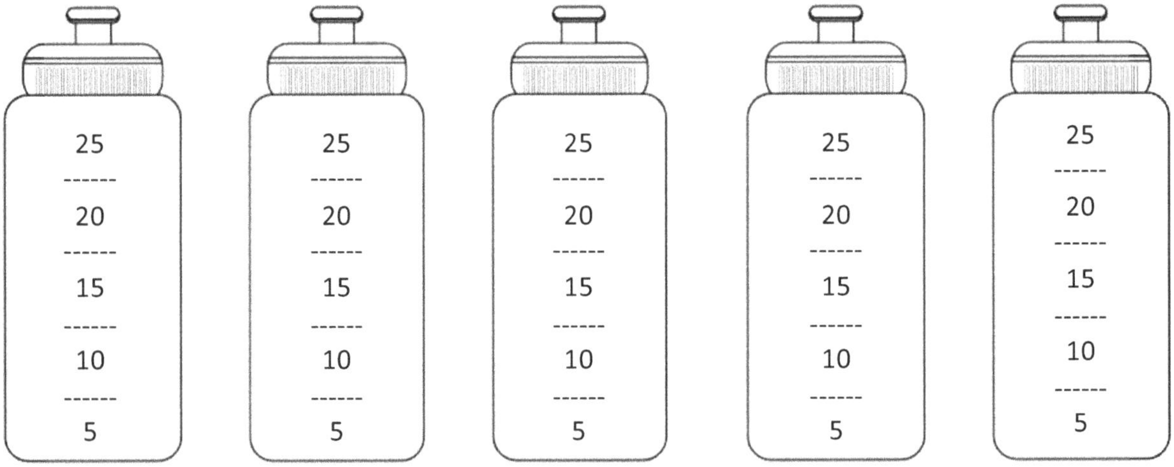

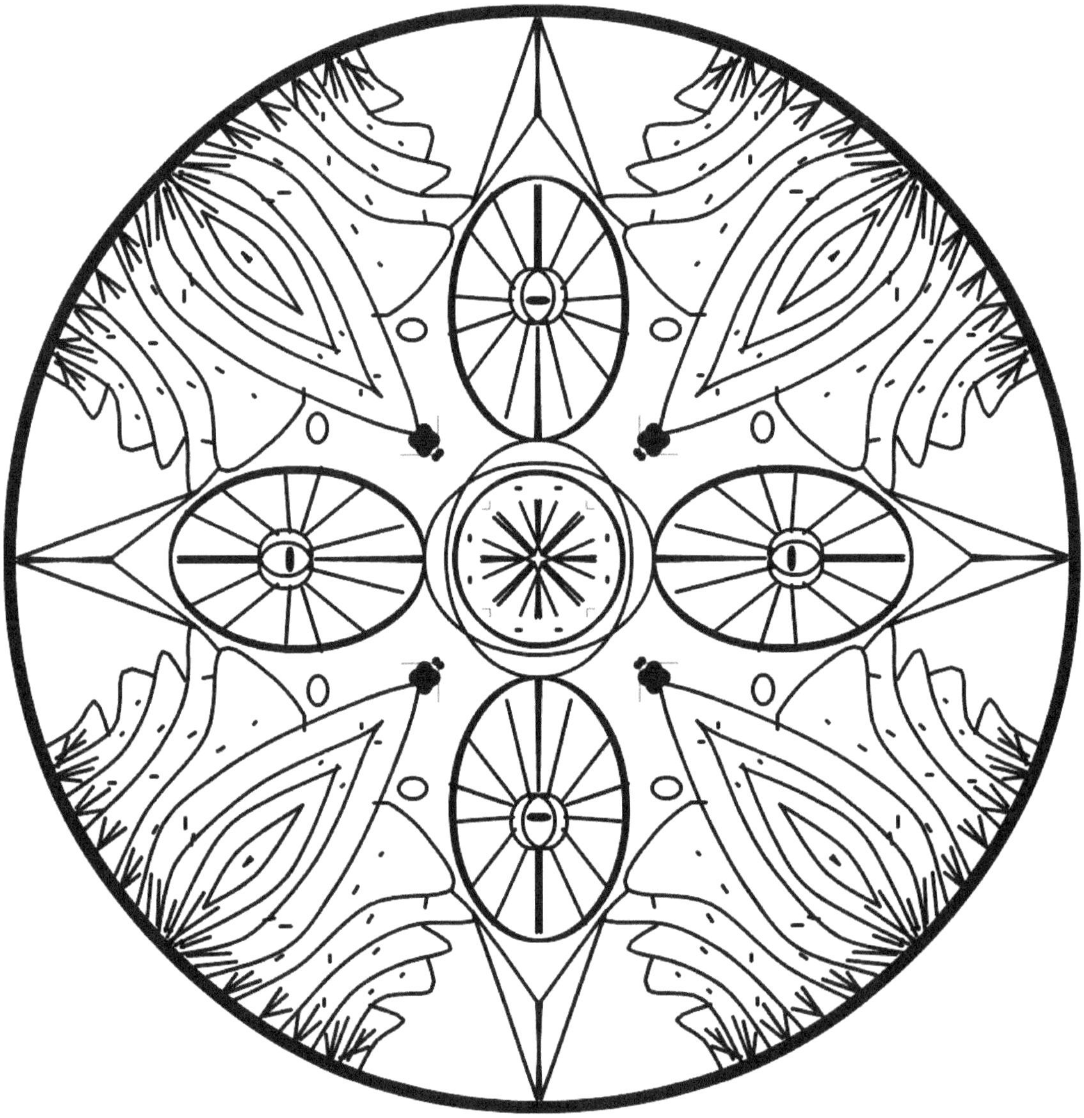

Measurements

DATE: ____________

Weight: _______

Neck _______

Shoulders _______

Chest _______

Bicep / upper arm left _________ right _______

Forearm left _________ right _______

Waist _______

Hips _______

Thighs left _________ right _____

Calf left _________ right _______

The Struggle You Are In Today, Is Developing The Strength You Need for Tomorrow.

Day Eleven ______

5:00 _______________________

6:00 _______________________

7:00 _______________________

8:00 _______________________

9:00 _______________________

10:00 _____________________

11:00 _____________________

Noon ______________________

1:00 _______________________

2:00 _______________________

3:00 _______________________

4:00 _______________________

5:00 _______________________

6:00 _______________________

7:00 _______________________

8:00 _______________________

9:00 _______________________

10:00 _____________________

11:00 _____________________

Midnight ___________________

top priorities for today

Today's victories

Give out as many hugs as you can today. How many did you give?

The Training

Exercise	Set 1	Set 2	Set 3	Set 4	Set 5	notes

Time started: _____________ Time ended: _____________

Location: ____

Feelings before training:

Feelings after training

NUTRITION

Meal 1

time eaten: _________

Meal 2

time eaten: _________

Meal 3

time eaten: _________

Meal 4

time eaten: _________

Meal 5

time eaten: _________

Hydration

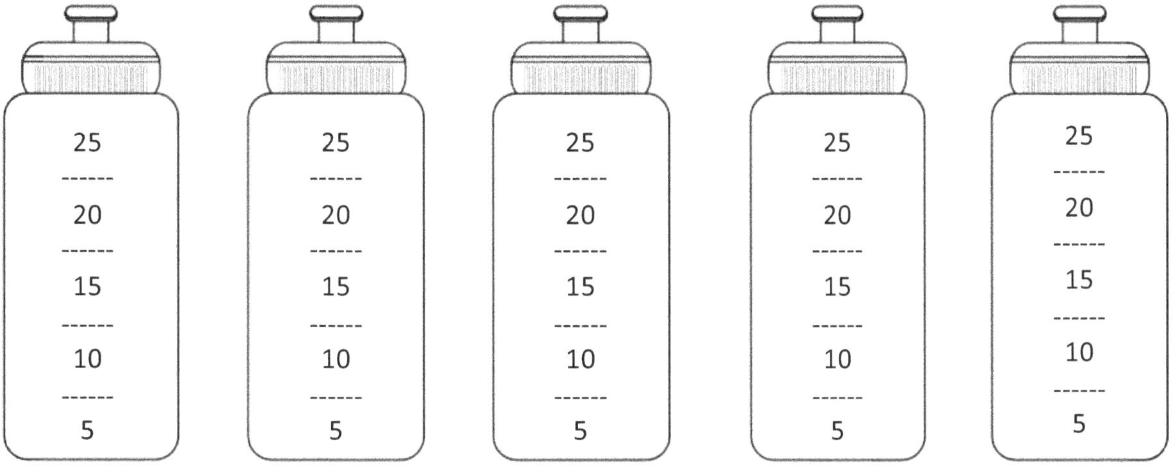

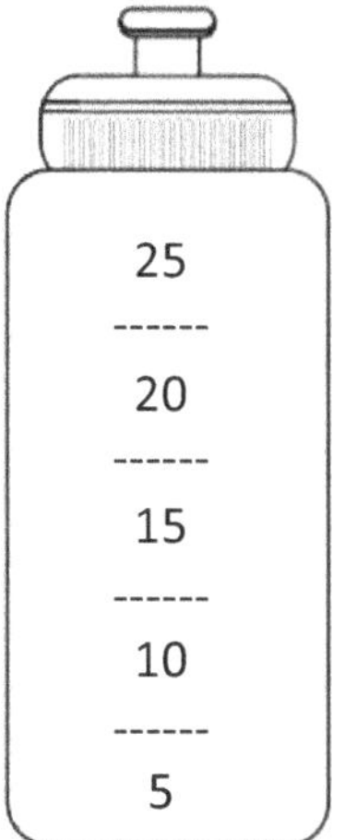 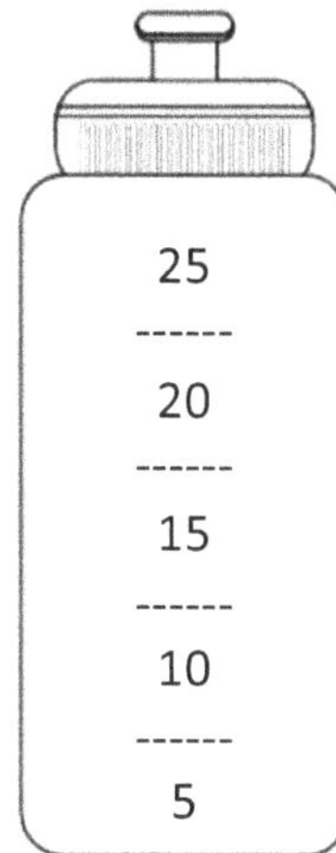

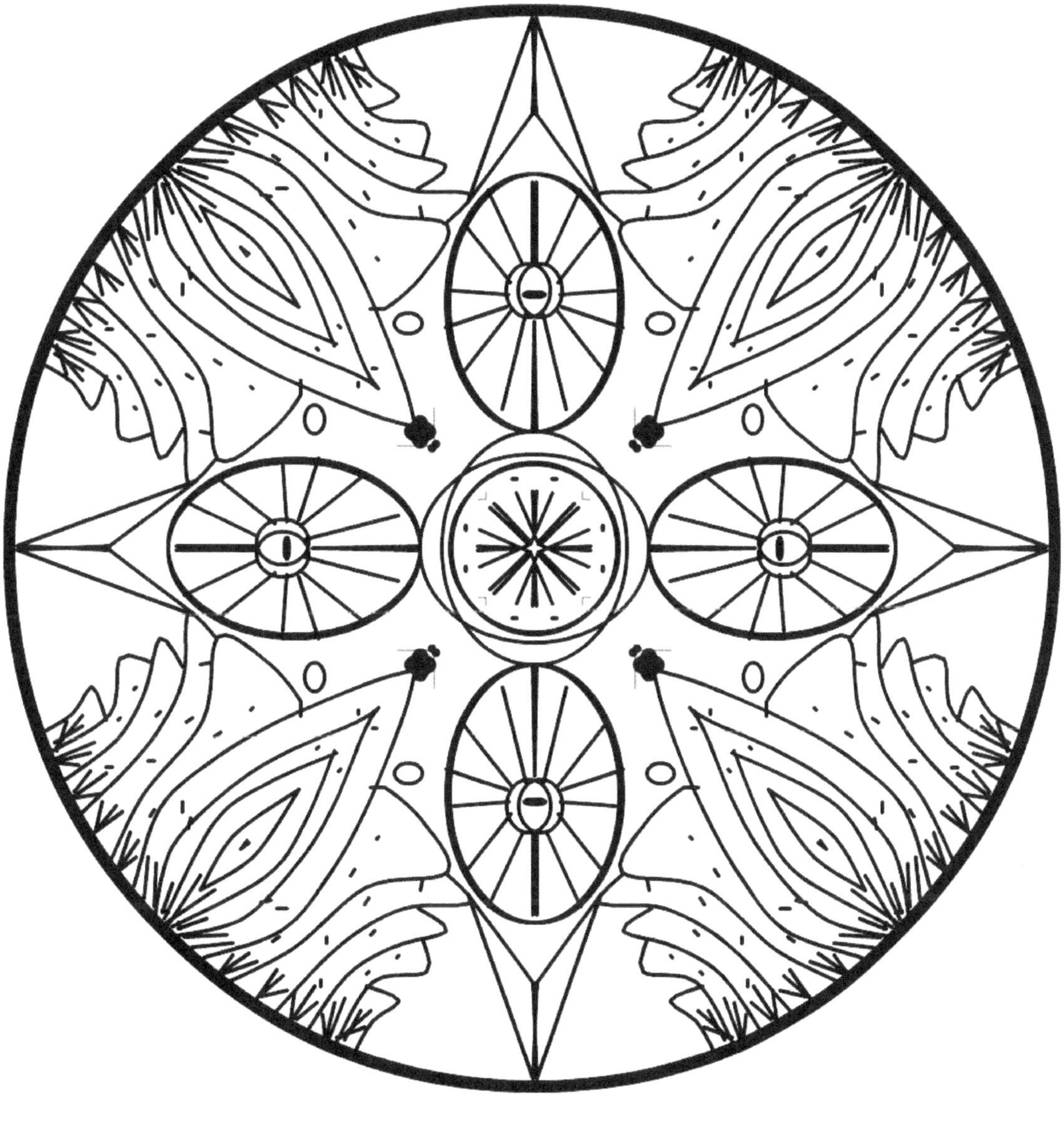

Day Twelve _______

5:00 _______________________

6:00 _______________________

7:00 _______________________

8:00 _______________________

9:00 _______________________

10:00 ______________________

11:00 ______________________

Noon _______________________

1:00 _______________________

2:00 _______________________

3:00 _______________________

4:00 _______________________

5:00 _______________________

6:00 _______________________

7:00 _______________________

8:00 _______________________

9:00 _______________________

10:00 ______________________

11:00 ______________________

Midnight ___________________

____

____

____

____

____

Today's victories

List 4 ways you show compassion.

____

____

____

____

____

____

The *Stella Society* Training

Exercise	Set 1	Set 2	Set 3	Set 4	Set 5	notes

Time started: _______________ Time ended: _______________

Location: ____

Feelings before training: 😊 😐 ☹ 😜 😠 🙁 😌 😎

Feelings after training 😊 😐 ☹ 😜 😠 🙁 😌 😎

NUTRITION

Meal 1

time eaten: _________

Meal 2

time eaten: _________

Meal 3

time eaten: _________

Meal 4

time eaten: _________

Meal 5

time eaten: _________

Hydration

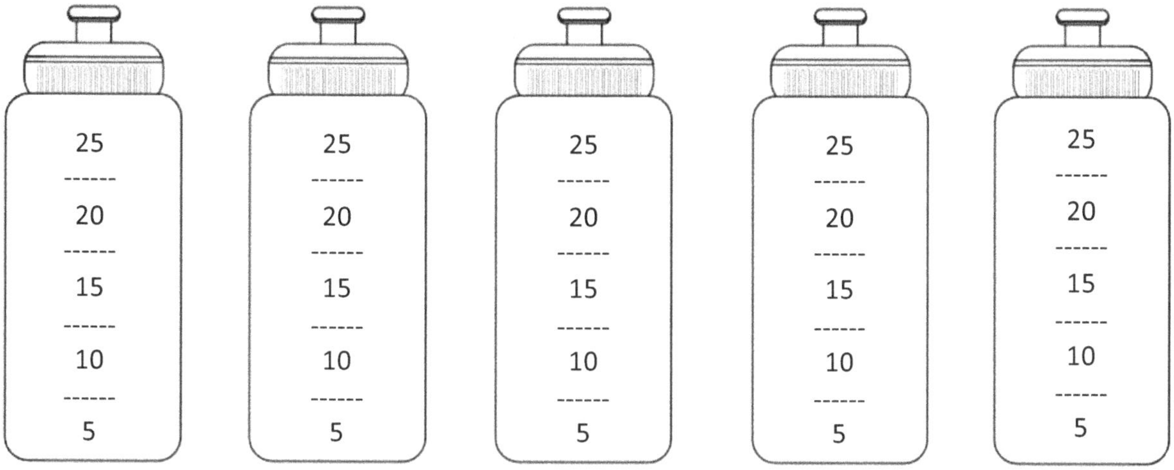

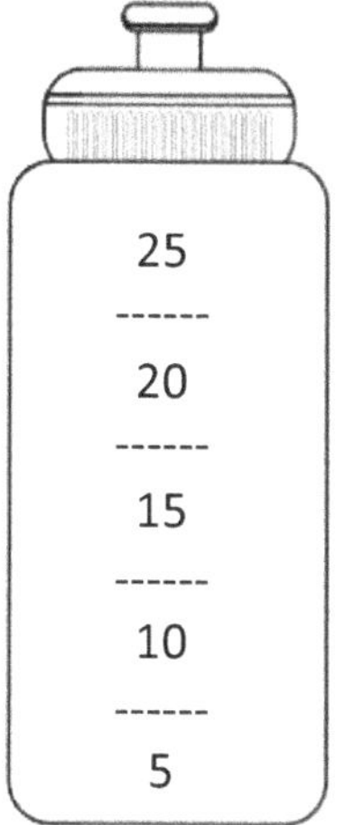

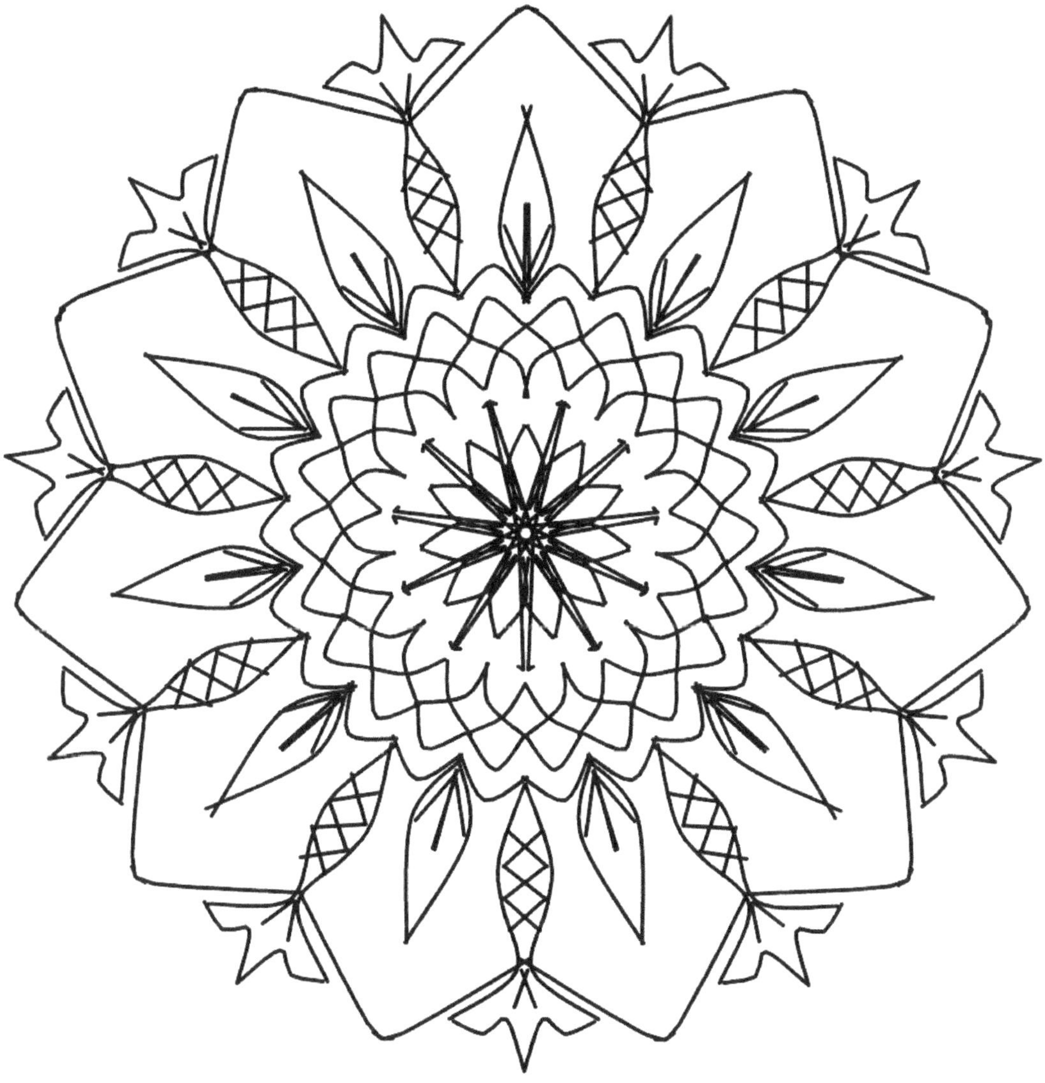

Day Thirteen _______

5:00 _________________	

5:00 _____________________

6:00 _____________________

7:00 _____________________

8:00 _____________________

9:00 _____________________

10:00 ____________________

11:00 ____________________

Noon _____________________

1:00 _____________________

2:00 _____________________

3:00 _____________________

4:00 _____________________

5:00 _____________________

6:00 _____________________

7:00 _____________________

8:00 _____________________

9:00 _____________________

10:00 ____________________

11:00 ____________________

Midnight _________________

top priorities for today 🎯

____

____

____

____

Today's victories 🏆

Who needs roses from your
garden and why?

____

____

____

____

____

____

The Stella Society Training

Exercise	Set 1	Set 2	Set 3	Set 4	Set 5	notes

Time started: _______________ Time ended: _______________

Location: ____

Feelings before training:        

Feelings after training        

NUTRITION

Meal 1

time eaten: _________

Meal 2

time eaten: _________

Meal 3

time eaten: _________

Meal 4

time eaten: _________

Meal 5

time eaten: _________

Hydration

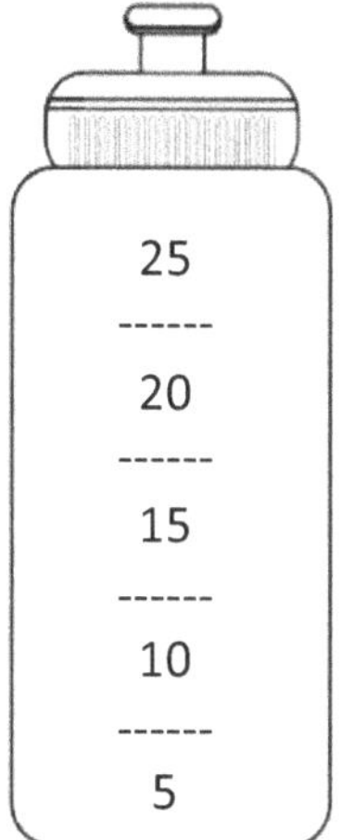
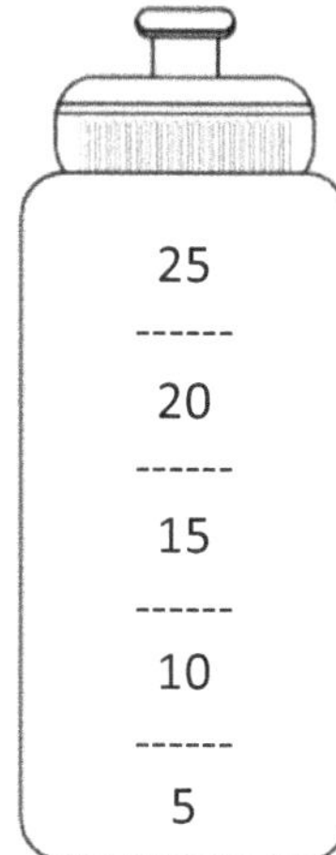
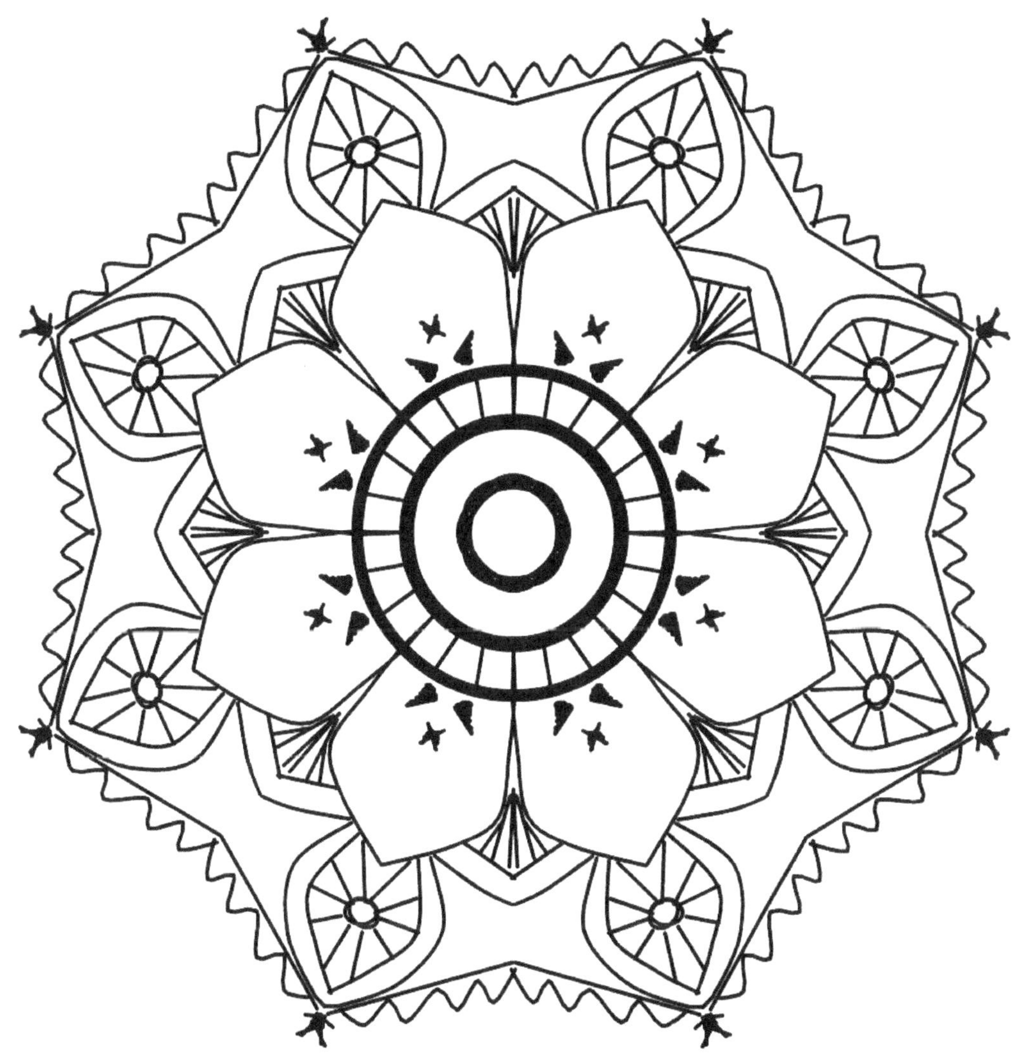

Day Fourteen _______

top priorities for today

____

____

____

____

____

Today's victories

What should you forgive
your self for?

____

____

____

____

____

____

The Stella Society Training

Exercise	Set 1	Set 2	Set 3	Set 4	Set 5	notes

Time started: ______________ Time ended: ______________

Location: ____

Feelings before training:        

Feelings after training        

NUTRITION

Meal 1

time eaten: _________

Meal 2

time eaten: _________

Meal 3

time eaten: _________

Meal 4

time eaten: _________

Meal 5

time eaten: _________

Hydration

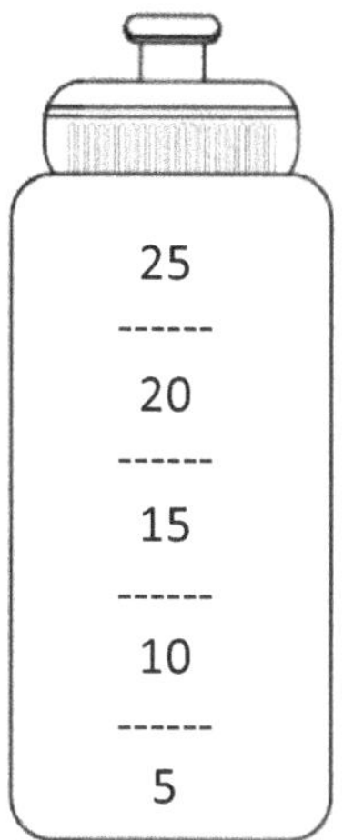

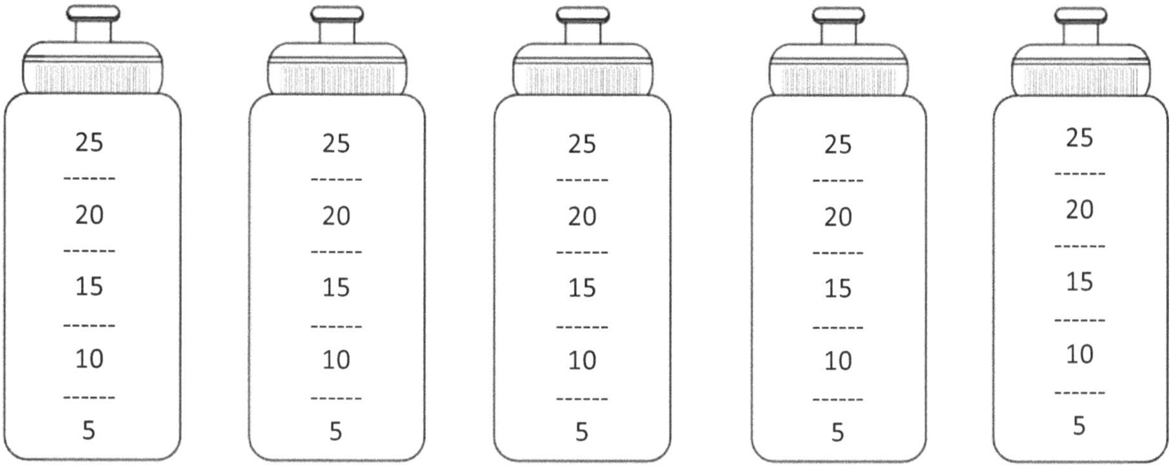

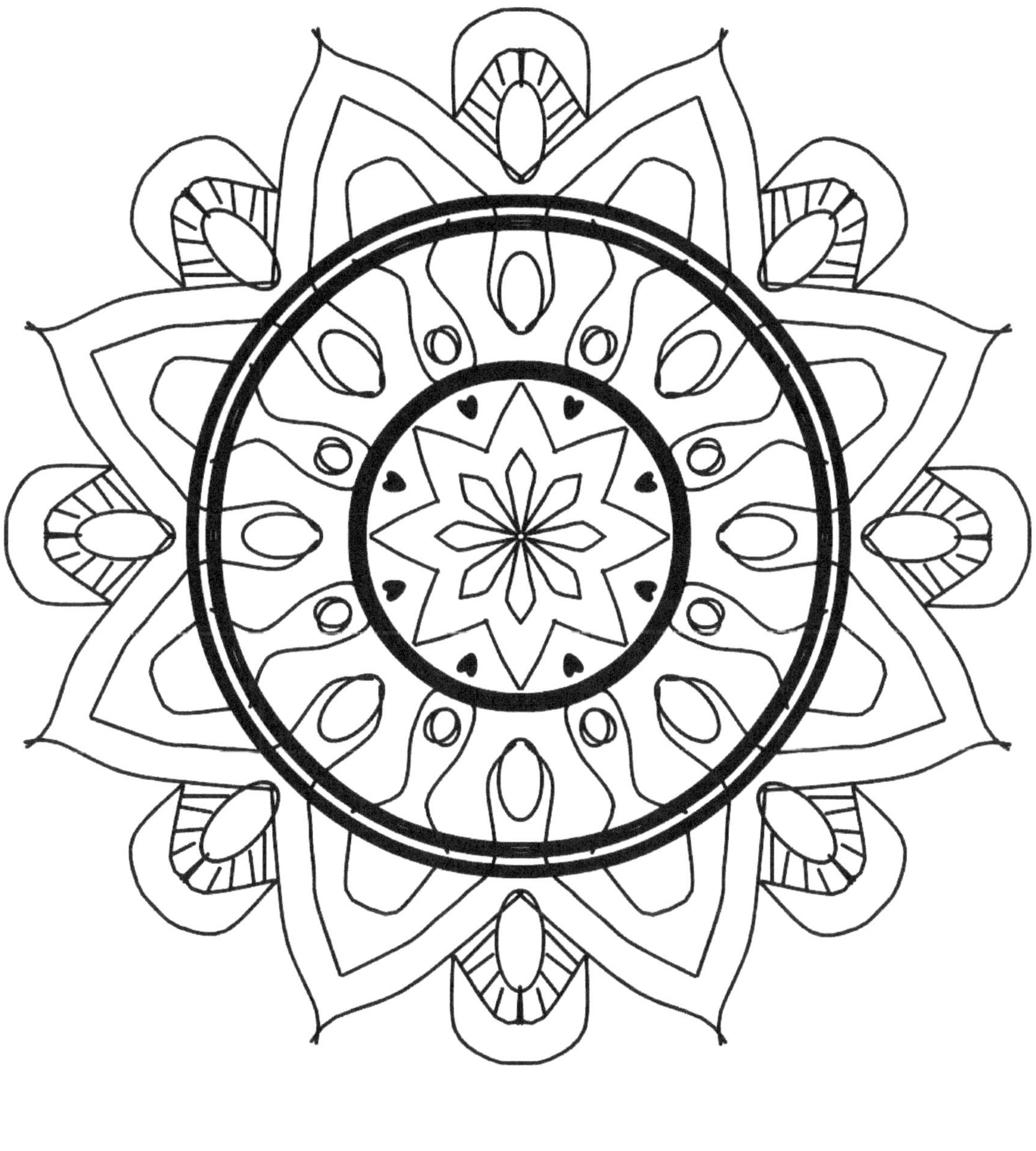

25	25	25	25	25
------	------	------	------	------
20	20	20	20	20
------	------	------	------	------
15	15	15	15	15
------	------	------	------	------
10	10	10	10	10
------	------	------	------	------
5	5	5	5	5

Day Fifteen _______

5:00 _______________________

6:00 _______________________

7:00 _______________________

8:00 _______________________

9:00 _______________________

10:00 ______________________

11:00 ______________________

Noon _______________________

1:00 _______________________

2:00 _______________________

3:00 _______________________

4:00 _______________________

5:00 _______________________

6:00 _______________________

7:00 _______________________

8:00 _______________________

9:00 _______________________

10:00 ______________________

11:00 ______________________

Midnight ___________________

top priorities for today

____

____

____

____

Today's victories

How will you be remarkable today?

____

____

____

____

____

____

The Stella Society Training

Exercise	Set 1	Set 2	Set 3	Set 4	Set 5	notes

Time started: _____________ Time ended: ______________

Location: ____

Feelings before training:        

Feelings after training        

NUTRITION

Meal 1

time eaten: _________

Meal 2

time eaten: _________

Meal 3

time eaten: _________

Meal 4

time eaten: _________

Meal 5

time eaten: _________

Hydration

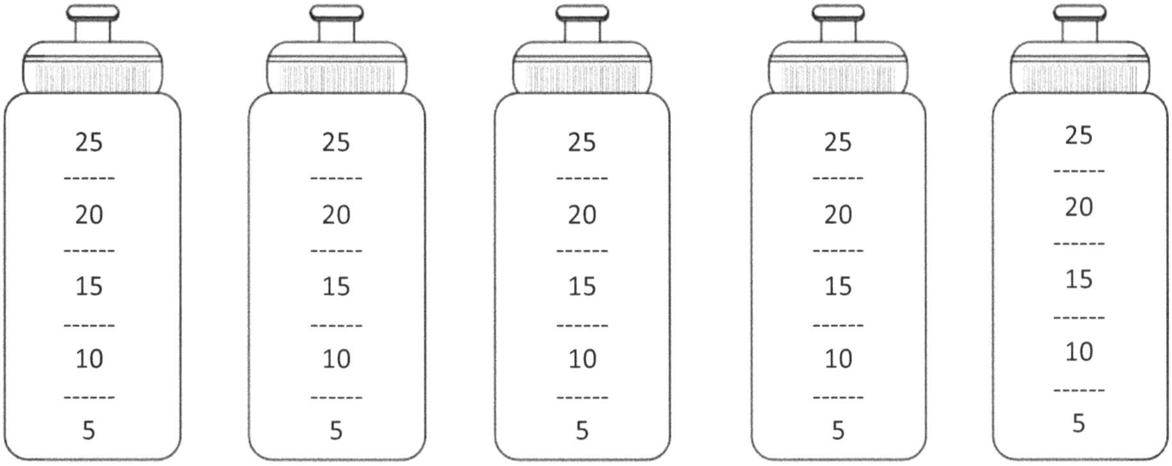

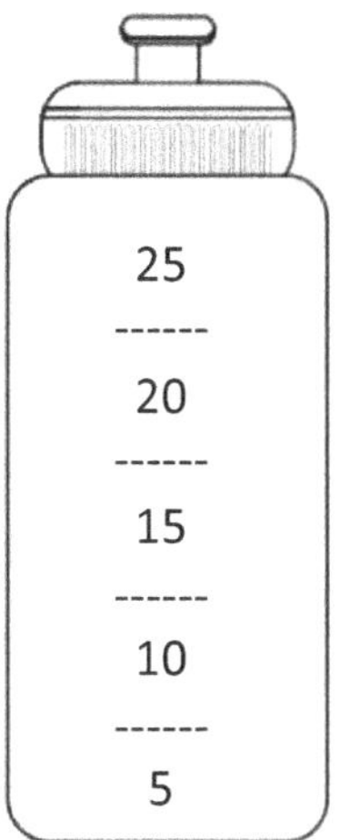

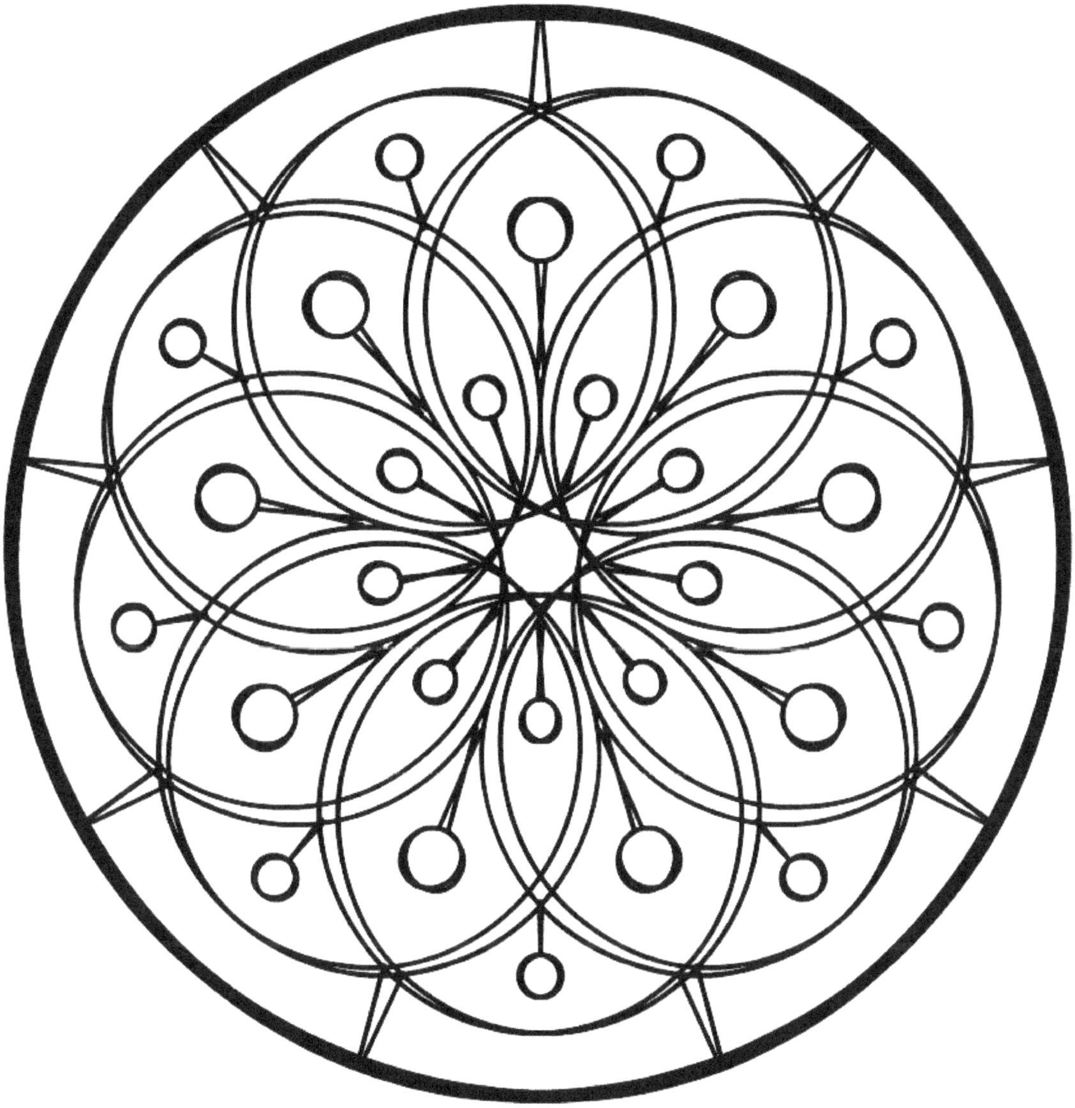

Day Sixteen _______

5:00 ______________________

6:00 ______________________

7:00 ______________________

8:00 ______________________

9:00 ______________________

10:00 _____________________

11:00 _____________________

Noon _____________________

1:00 ______________________

2:00 ______________________

3:00 ______________________

4:00 ______________________

5:00 ______________________

6:00 ______________________

7:00 ______________________

8:00 ______________________

9:00 ______________________

10:00 _____________________

11:00 _____________________

Midnight __________________

top priorities for today

____

____

____

____

Today's victories

Watch the sunset and list 5 places you want to see it happen?

____

____

____

____

____

____

The Training

Exercise	Set 1	Set 2	Set 3	Set 4	Set 5	notes

Time started: ______________ Time ended: _______________

Location: ____

Feelings before training:

Feelings after training

NUTRITION

Meal 1

time eaten: _________

Meal 2

time eaten: _________

Meal 3

time eaten: _________

Meal 4

time eaten: _________

Meal 5

time eaten: _________

Hydration

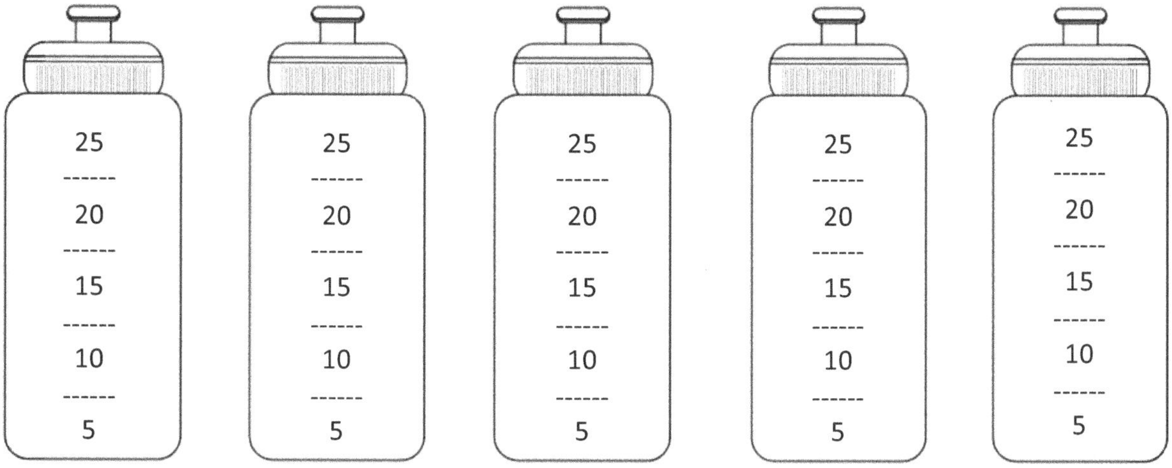

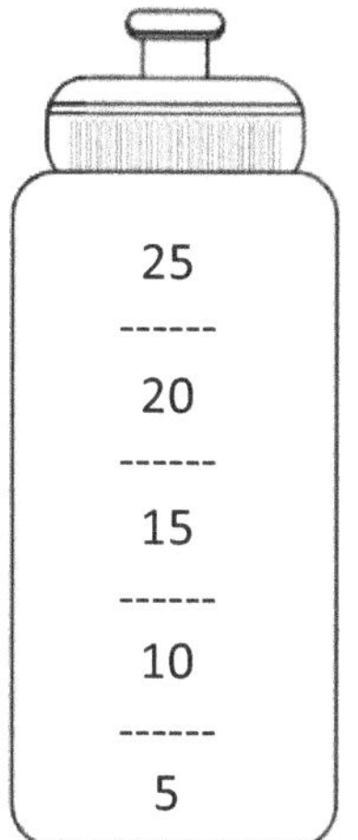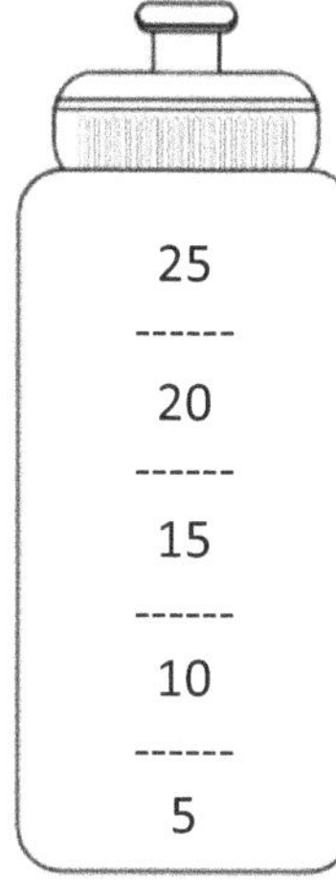

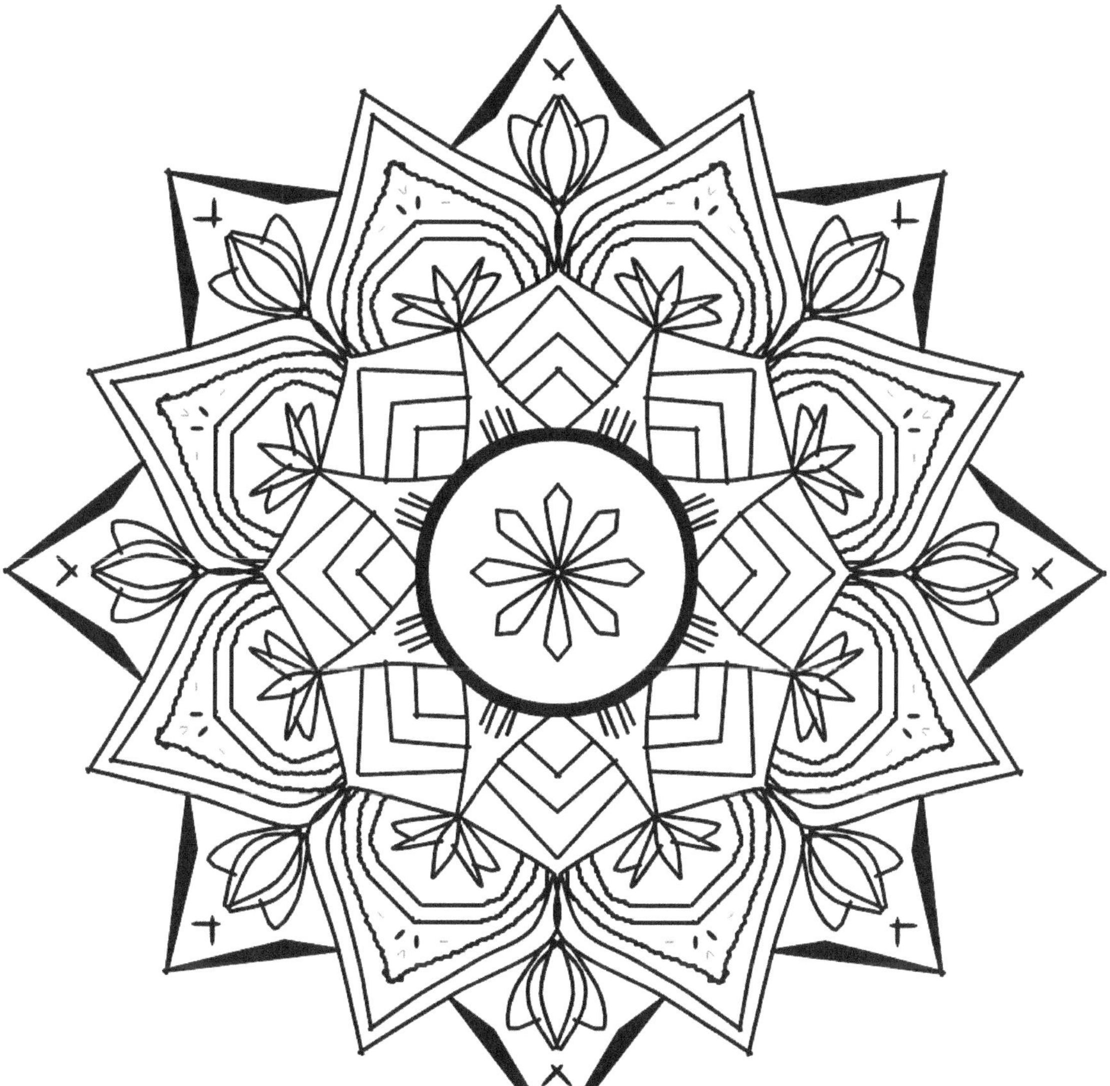

Day Seventeen __________

5:00 __________________________

6:00 __________________________

7:00 __________________________

8:00 __________________________

9:00 __________________________

10:00 _________________________

11:00 _________________________

Noon __________________________

1:00 __________________________

2:00 __________________________

3:00 __________________________

4:00 __________________________

5:00 __________________________

6:00 __________________________

7:00 __________________________

8:00 __________________________

9:00 __________________________

10:00 _________________________

11:00 _________________________

Midnight ______________________

top priorities for today

____

____

____

____

Today's victories

What makes you happy?

____

____

____

____

____

____

The Stella Society Training

Exercise	Set 1	Set 2	Set 3	Set 4	Set 5	notes

Time started: _____________ Time ended: _____________

Location: ____

Feelings before training: 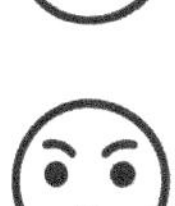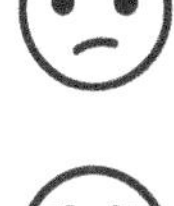

Feelings after training 

NUTRITION

Meal 1

time eaten: _________

Meal 2

time eaten: _________

Meal 3

time eaten: _________

Meal 4

time eaten: _________

Meal 5

time eaten: _________

Hydration

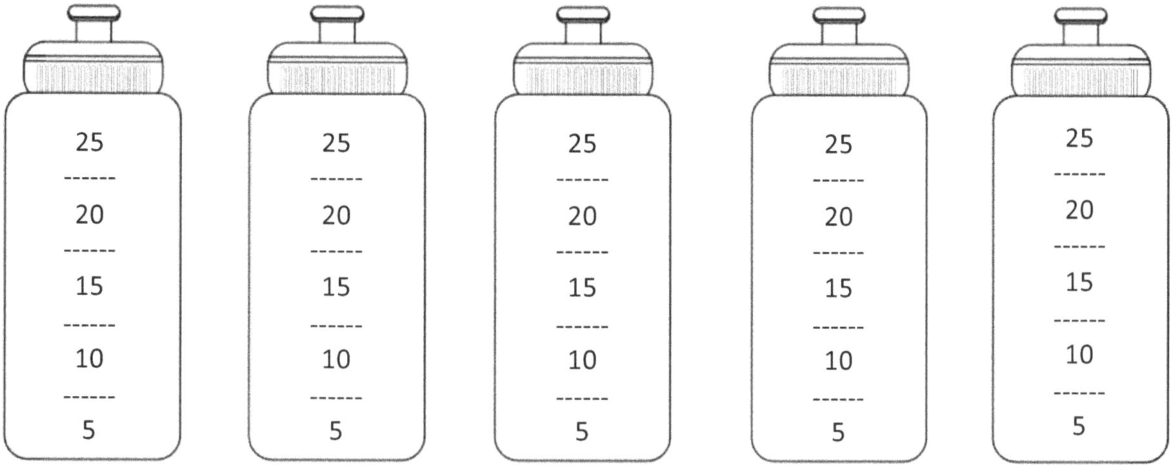

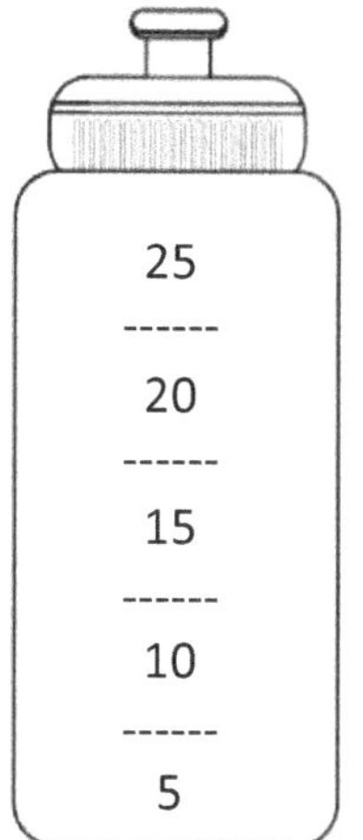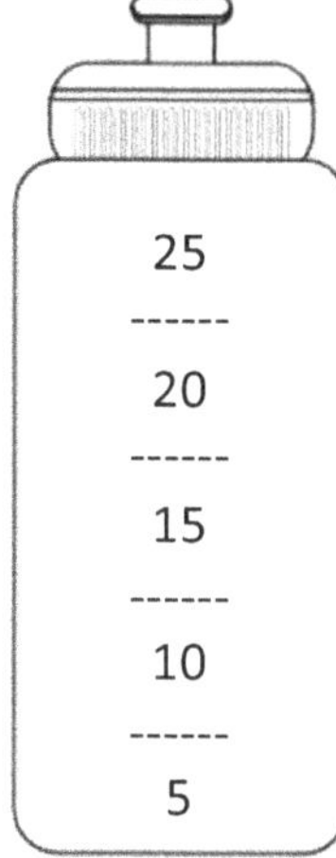

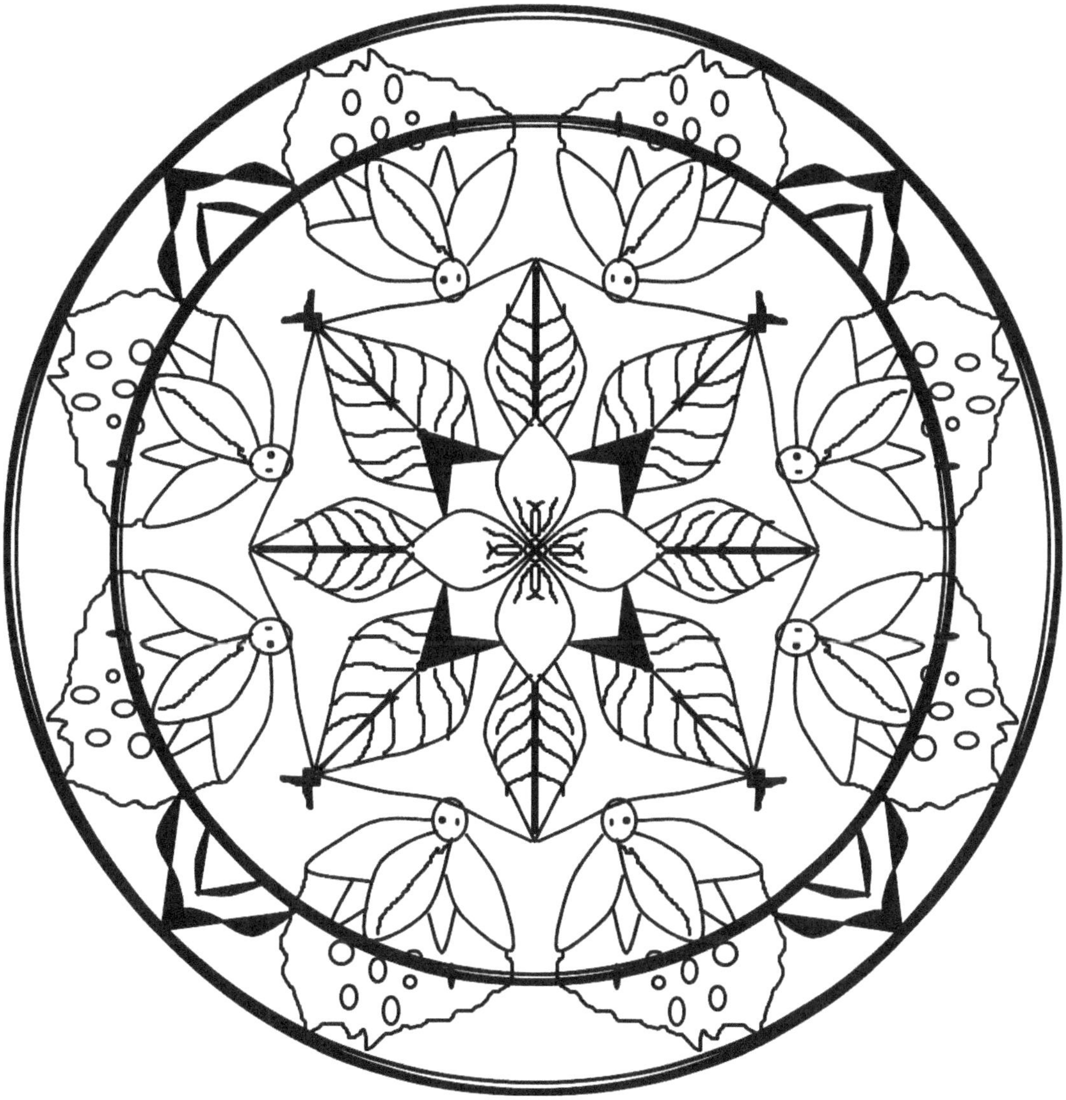

Day Eighteen _______

5:00 ______________________

6:00 ______________________

7:00 ______________________

8:00 ______________________

9:00 ______________________

10:00 ______________________

11:00 ______________________

Noon ______________________

1:00 ______________________

2:00 ______________________

3:00 ______________________

4:00 ______________________

5:00 ______________________

6:00 ______________________

7:00 ______________________

8:00 ______________________

9:00 ______________________

10:00 ______________________

11:00 ______________________

Midnight __________________

The ⚇ *Stella Society* Training

Exercise	Set 1	Set 2	Set 3	Set 4	Set 5	notes

Time started: _____________   Time ended: _____________

Location: ____

Feelings before training: 🙂 😐 ☹️ 😜 😠 😕 😇 😎

Feelings after training 🙂 😐 ☹️ 😜 😠 😕 😇 😎

NUTRITION

Meal 1

time eaten: _________

Meal 2

time eaten: _________

Meal 3

time eaten: _________

Meal 4

time eaten: _________

Meal 5

time eaten: _________

Hydration

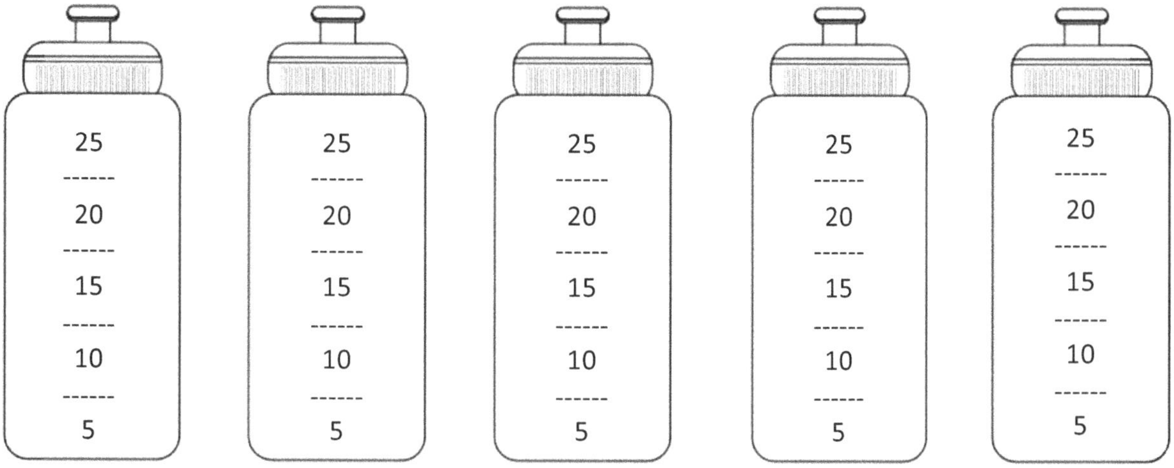

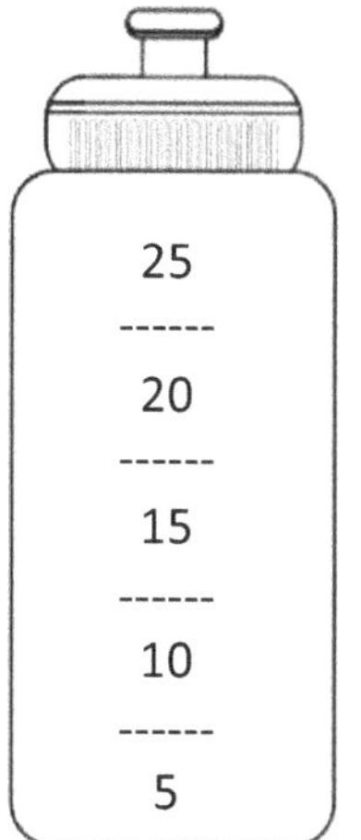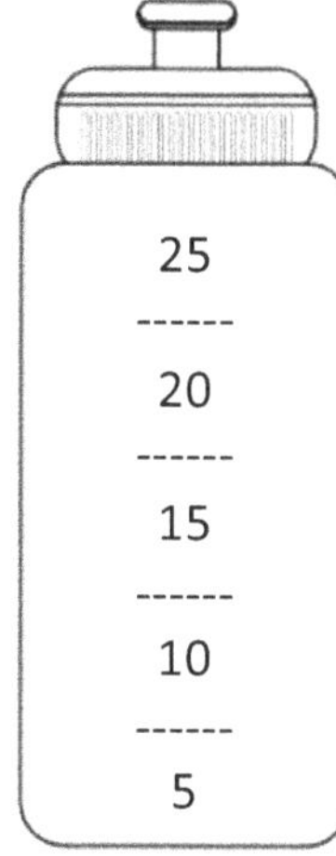

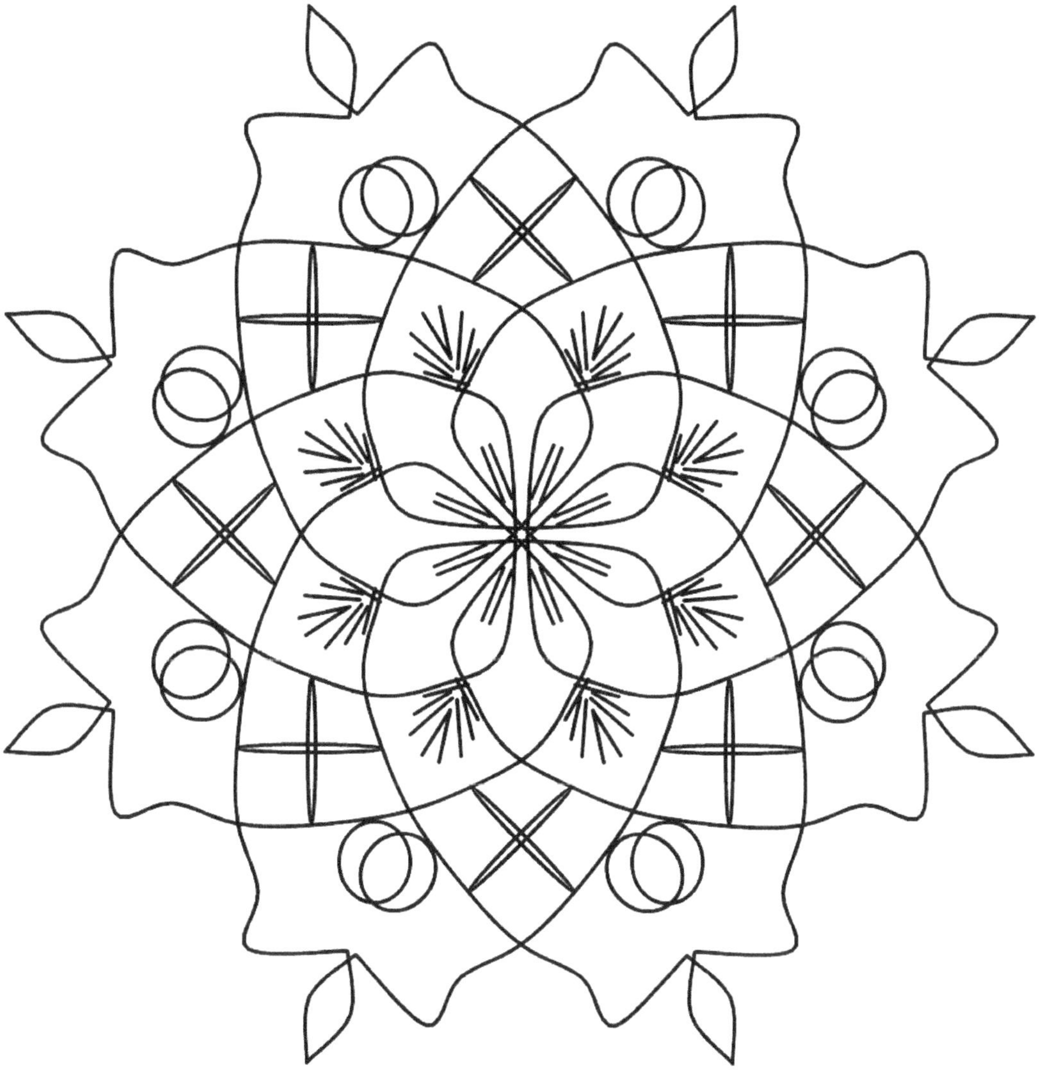

Day Nineteen _______

5:00 _______________________

6:00 _______________________

7:00 _______________________

8:00 _______________________

9:00 _______________________

10:00 _______________________

11:00 _______________________

Noon _______________________

1:00 _______________________

2:00 _______________________

3:00 _______________________

4:00 _______________________

5:00 _______________________

6:00 _______________________

7:00 _______________________

8:00 _______________________

9:00 _______________________

10:00 _______________________

11:00 _______________________

Midnight _______________________

top priorities for today

____

____

____

____

Today's victories

You are charming, how will you show it?

____

____

____

____

____

____

The Stella Society Training

Exercise	Set 1	Set 2	Set 3	Set 4	Set 5	notes

Time started: _______________ Time ended: _______________

Location: ____

Feelings before training:       

Feelings after training  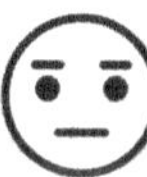      

NUTRITION

Meal 1

time eaten: _________

Meal 2

time eaten: _________

Meal 3

time eaten: _________

Meal 4

time eaten: _________

Meal 5

time eaten: _________

Hydration

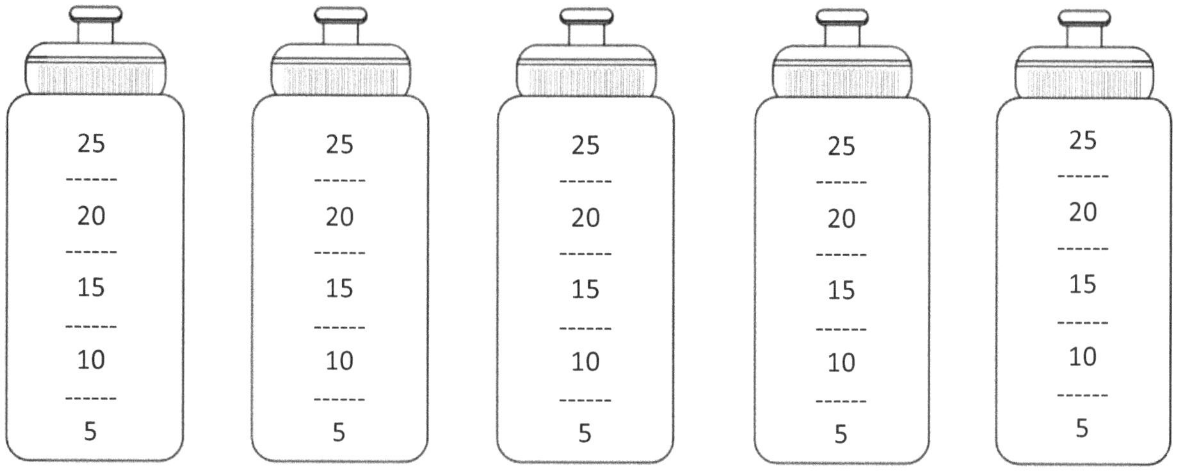

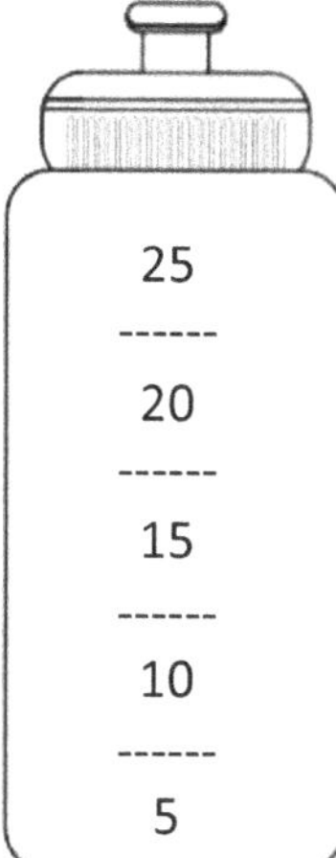 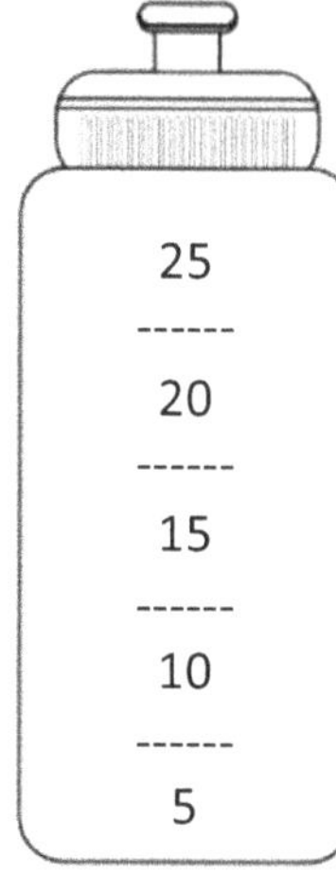

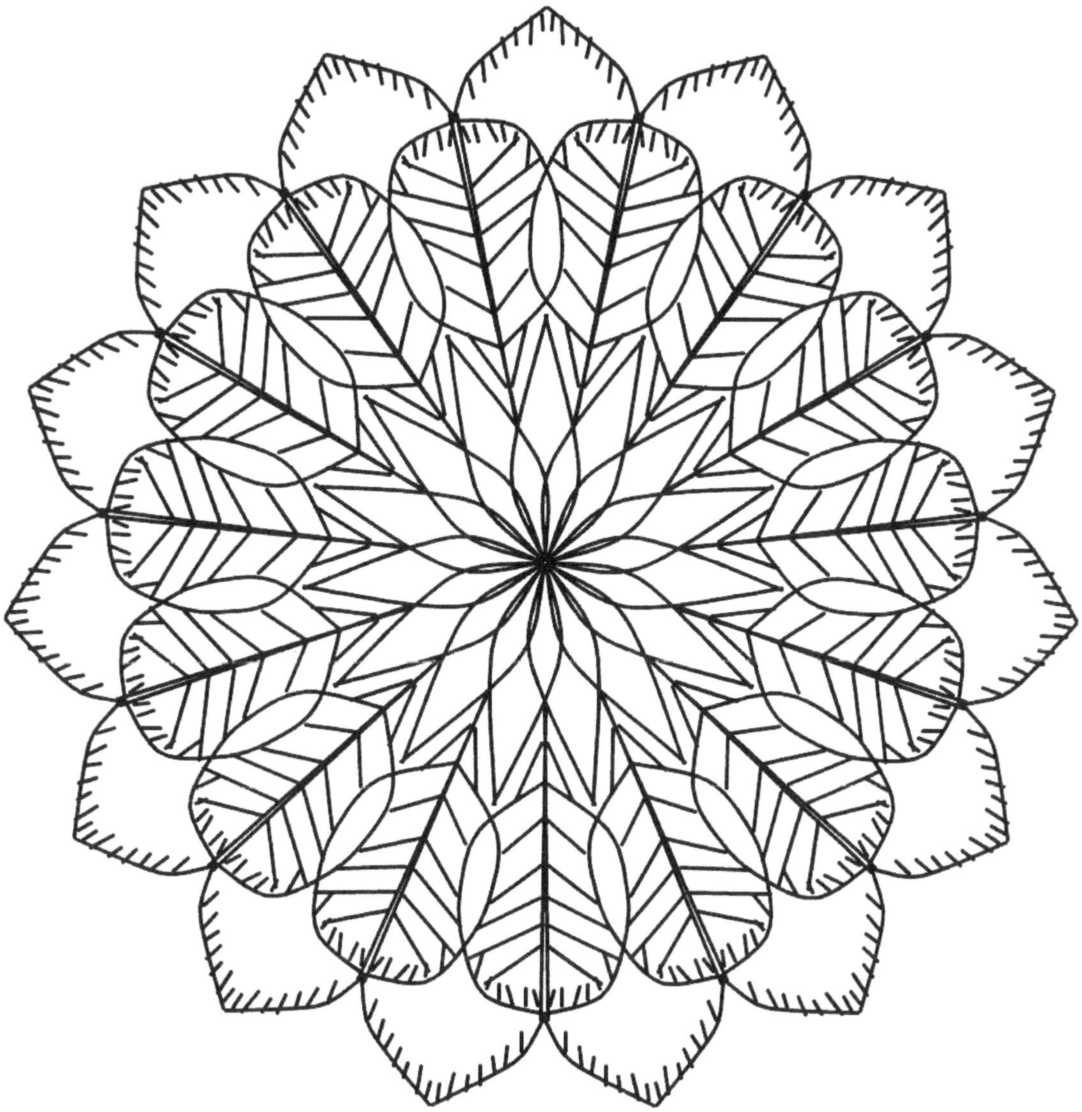

Measurements

DATE: _________

P

Weight: ______

R

Neck ______

O

Shoulders ______

Chest ______

G

Bicep / upper arm left ________ right _______

Forearm left ________ right ______

R

Waist ______

Hips ______

E

Thighs left _______ right ______

S

Calf left ________ right _______

S

(vertical right margin: C H E C K)

Food, Like Your Money,
Should Be Working For You

Day Twenty _______

5:00	_______________________
6:00	_______________________
7:00	_______________________
8:00	_______________________
9:00	_______________________
10:00	_______________________
11:00	_______________________
Noon	_______________________
1:00	_______________________
2:00	_______________________
3:00	_______________________
4:00	_______________________
5:00	_______________________
6:00	_______________________
7:00	_______________________
8:00	_______________________
9:00	_______________________
10:00	_______________________
11:00	_______________________
Midnight	_______________________

top priorities for today

____
____
____
____

Today's victories

What is your level of understanding difficult situations?

____
____
____
____

The *Stella Society* Workout

Exercise	Set 1	Set 2	Set 3	Set 4	Set 5	notes

Time started: ______________ Time ended: _______________

Location: ____

Feelings before training: 😊 😐 🙁 😜 😠 😟 😊 😎

Feelings after training 😊 😐 🙁 😜 😠 😟 😊 😎

NUTRITION

Meal 1

time eaten: _________

Meal 2

time eaten: _________

Meal 3

time eaten: _________

Meal 4

time eaten: _________

Meal 5

time eaten: _________

Hydration

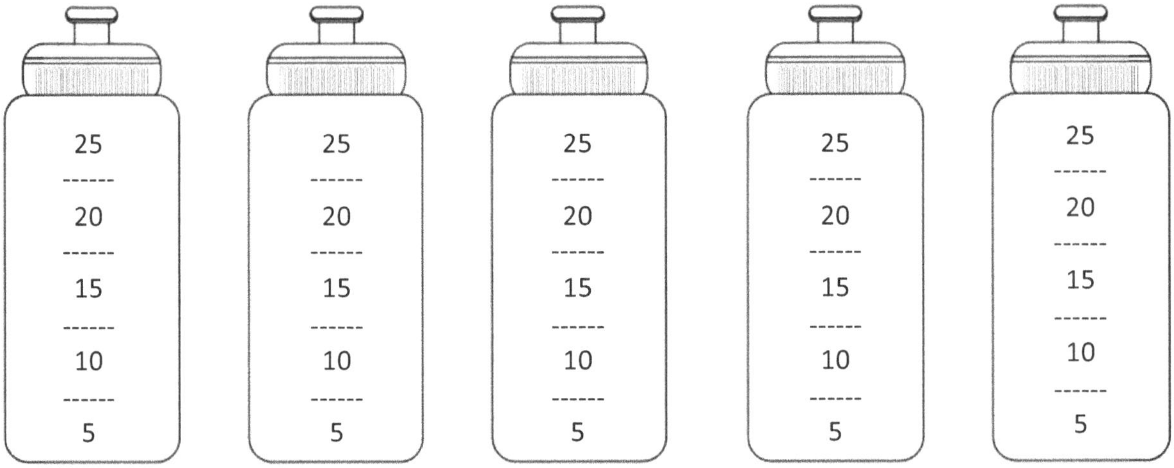

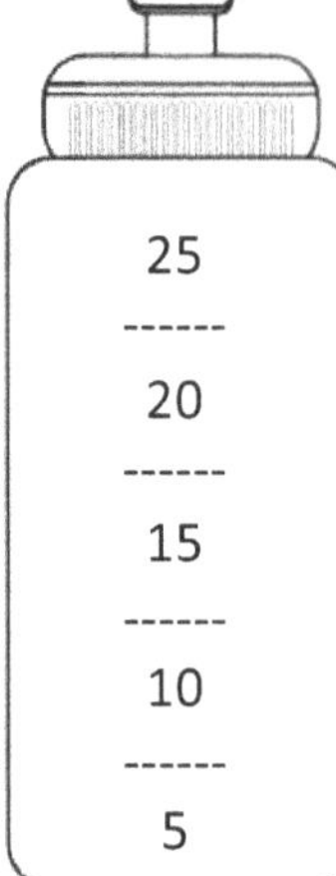

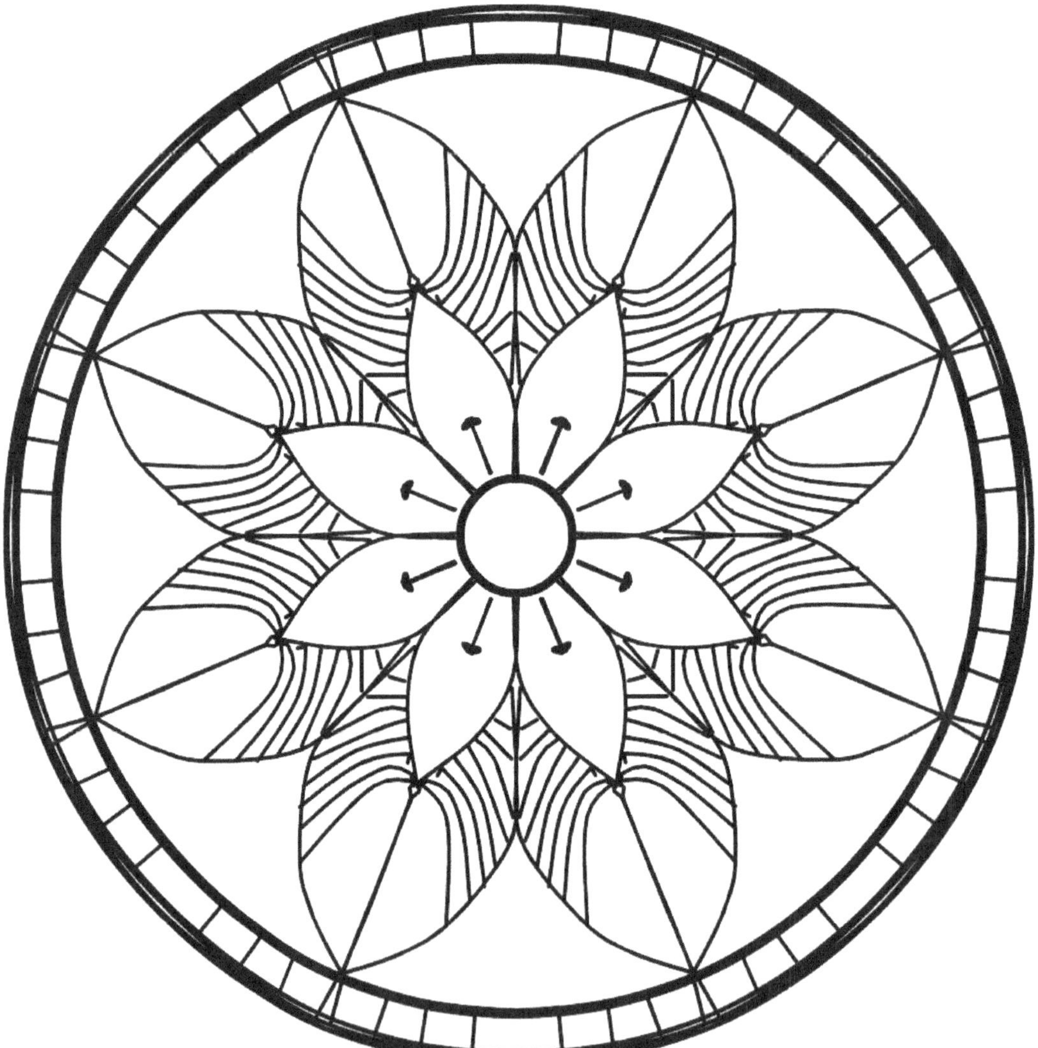

Day Twenty-one ______

5:00 ______________________

6:00 ______________________

7:00 ______________________

8:00 ______________________

9:00 ______________________

10:00 ____________________

11:00 ____________________

Noon _____________________

1:00 ______________________

2:00 ______________________

3:00 ______________________

4:00 ______________________

5:00 ______________________

6:00 ______________________

7:00 ______________________

8:00 ______________________

9:00 ______________________

10:00 ____________________

11:00 ____________________

Midnight __________________

top priorities for today

Today's victories

How much can you endure?

The Stella Society Workout

Exercise	Set 1	Set 2	Set 3	Set 4	Set 5	notes

Time started: _______________   Time ended: _______________

Location: ____

Feelings before training:        

Feelings after training

NUTRITION

Meal 1
time eaten: _________

Meal 2
time eaten: _________

Meal 3
time eaten: _________

Meal 4
time eaten: _________

Meal 5
time eaten: _________

Hydration

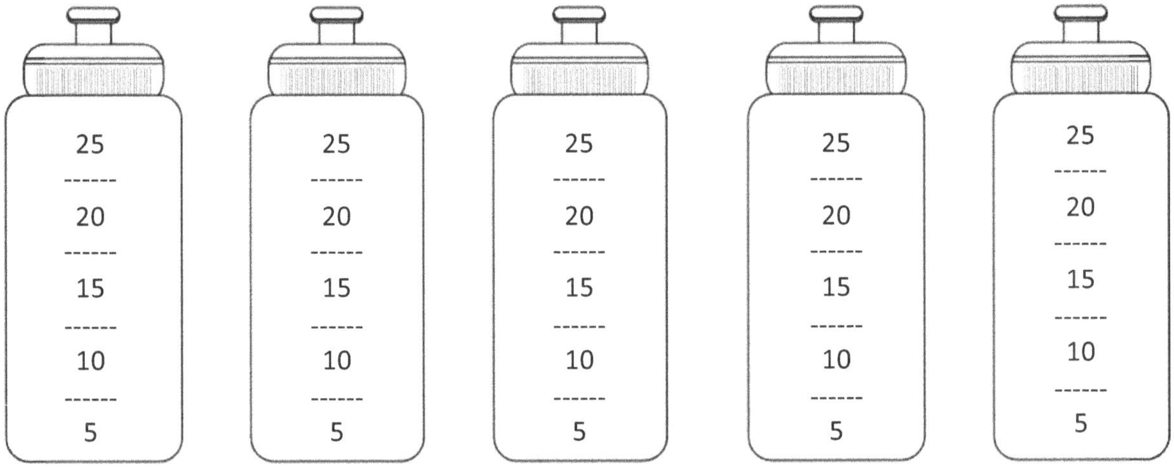

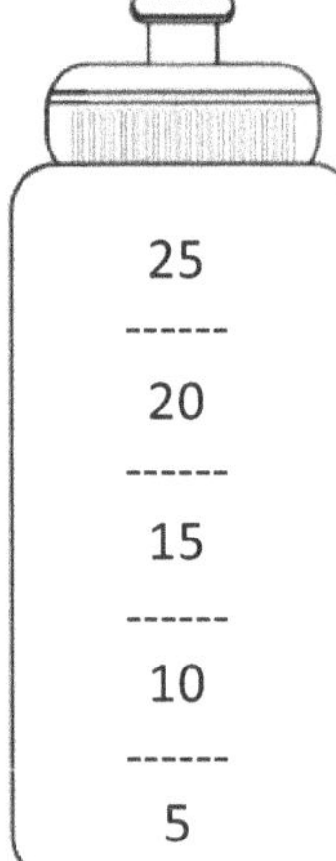

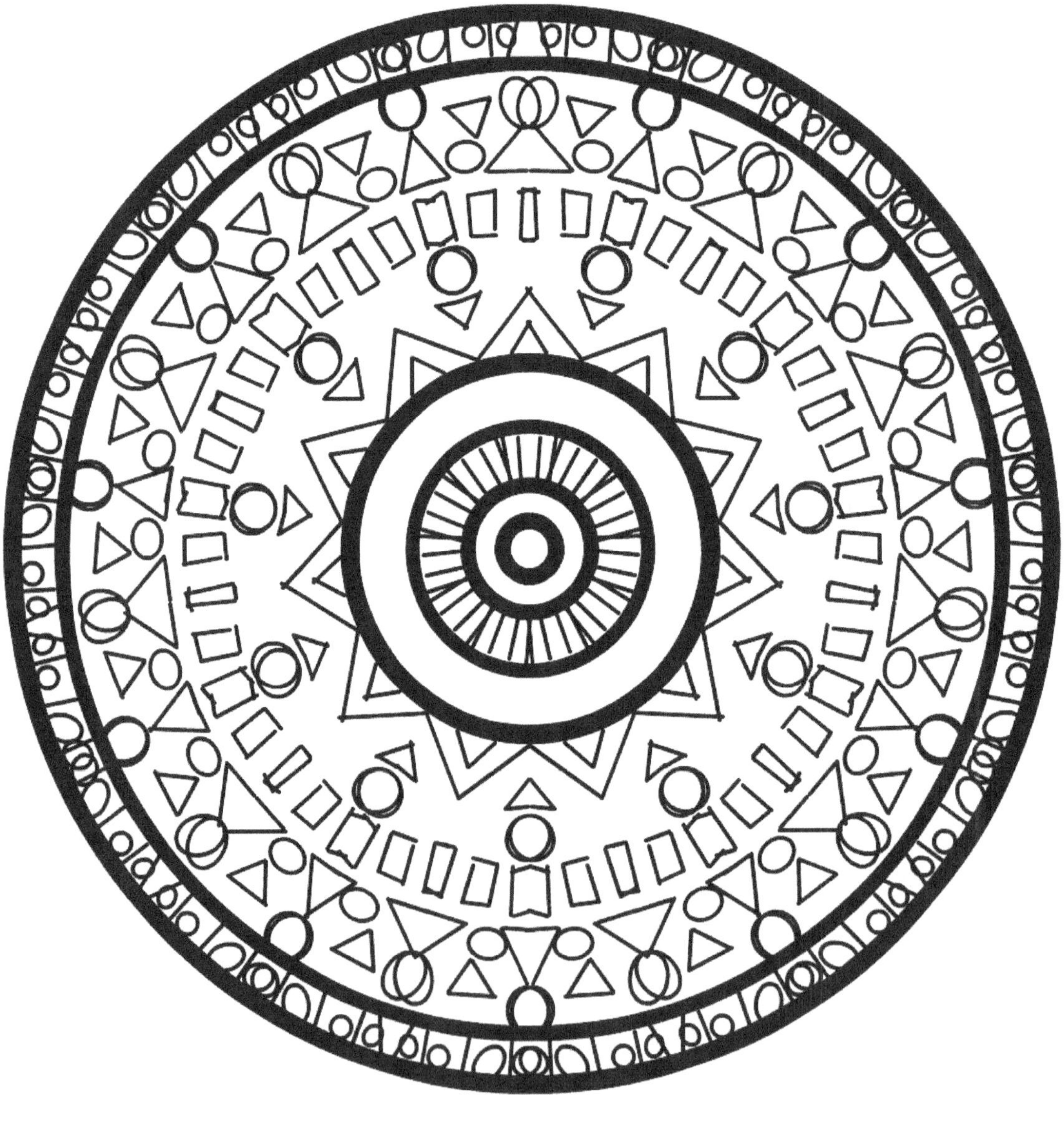

Day Twenty-two ______

5:00 ________________________

6:00 ________________________

7:00 ________________________

8:00 ________________________

9:00 ________________________

10:00 ________________________

11:00 ________________________

Noon ________________________

1:00 ________________________

2:00 ________________________

3:00 ________________________

4:00 ________________________

5:00 ________________________

6:00 ________________________

7:00 ________________________

8:00 ________________________

9:00 ________________________

10:00 ________________________

11:00 ________________________

Midnight ______________________

List 5 ways to be thoughtful.

The Stella Society Workout

Exercise	Set 1	Set 2	Set 3	Set 4	Set 5	notes

Time started: _____________ Time ended: _______________

Location: ____

Feelings before training: 🙂 😑 🙁 😜 😠 😟 😊 😎

Feelings after training 🙂 😑 🙁 😜 😠 😟 😊 😎

NUTRITION

Meal 1
time eaten: _________

Meal 2
time eaten: _________

Meal 3
time eaten: _________

Meal 4
time eaten: _________

Meal 5
time eaten: _________

Hydration

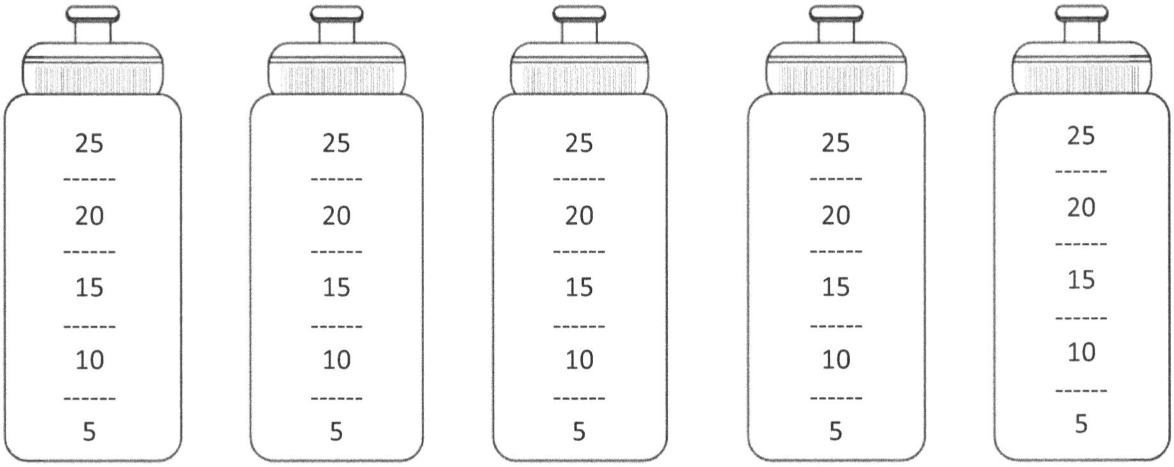

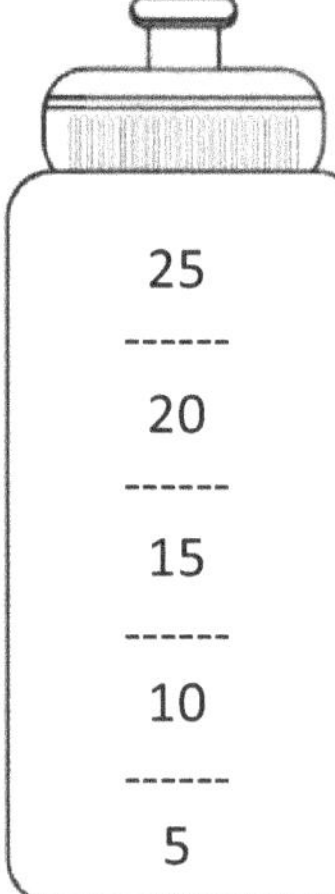

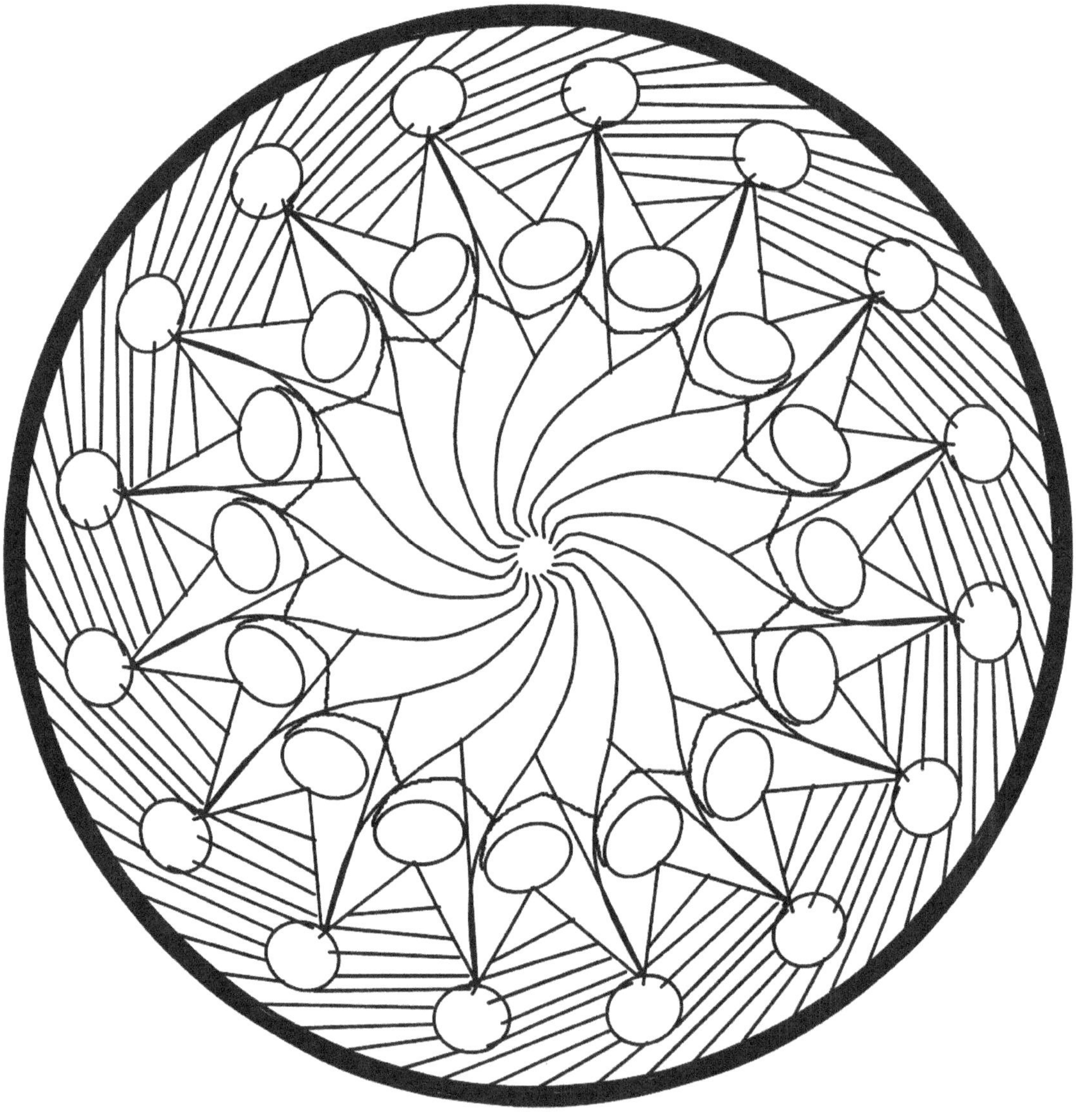

Day Twenty-three _______

5:00 _______________________

6:00 _______________________

7:00 _______________________

8:00 _______________________

9:00 _______________________

10:00 _______________________

11:00 _______________________

Noon _______________________

1:00 _______________________

2:00 _______________________

3:00 _______________________

4:00 _______________________

5:00 _______________________

6:00 _______________________

7:00 _______________________

8:00 _______________________

9:00 _______________________

10:00 _______________________

11:00 _______________________

Midnight _____________________

top priorities for today

____

____

____

____

Today's victories

Why should you be unapologetic?

____

____

____

____

____

____

The *Stella Society* Workout

Exercise	Set 1	Set 2	Set 3	Set 4	Set 5	notes

Time started: _____________   Time ended: ______________

Location: ____

Feelings before training: 🙂 😐 🙁 😜 😣 😟 😊 😎

Feelings after training 🙂 😐 🙁 😜 😣 😟 😊 😎

NUTRITION

Meal 1
time eaten: _________

Meal 2
time eaten: _________

Meal 3
time eaten: _________

Meal 4
time eaten: _________

Meal 5
time eaten: _________

Hydration

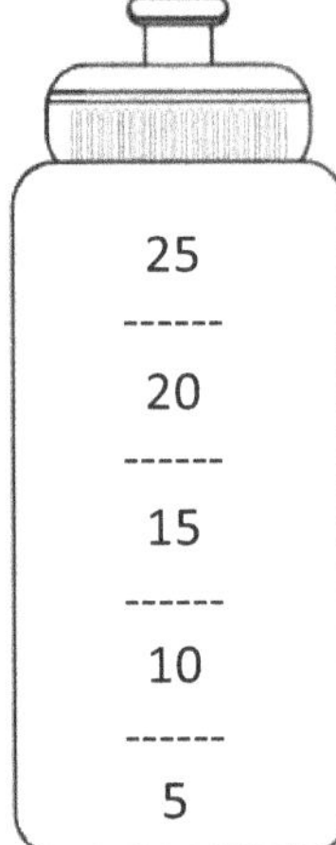
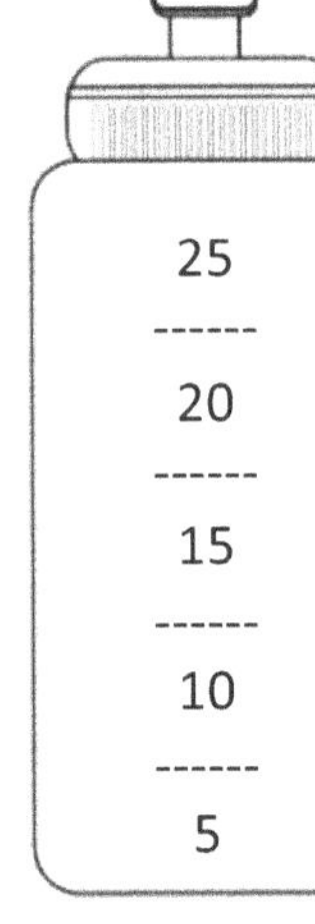
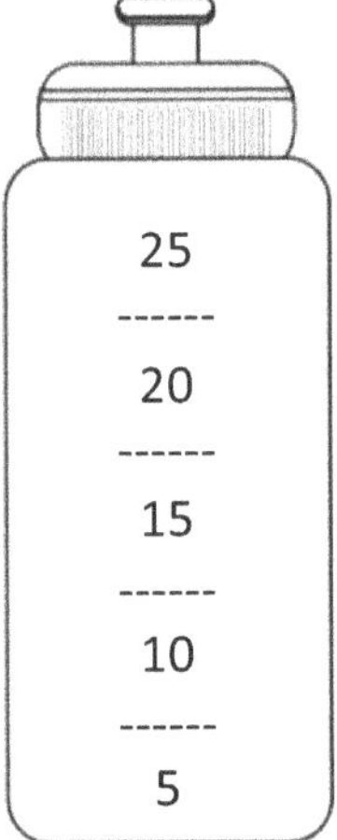
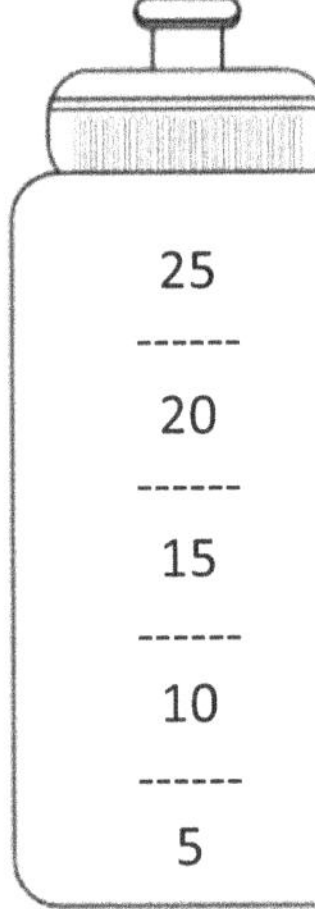
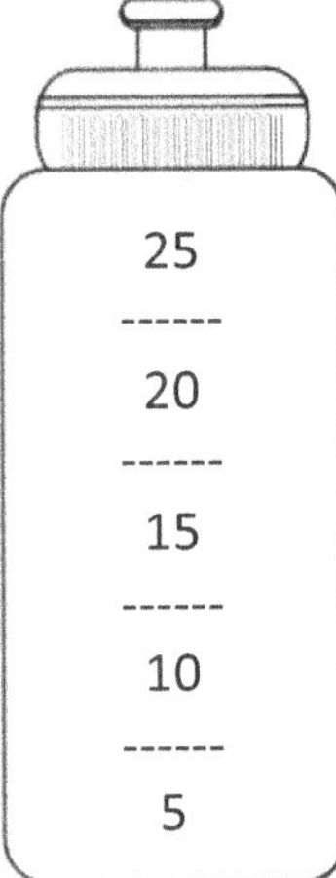

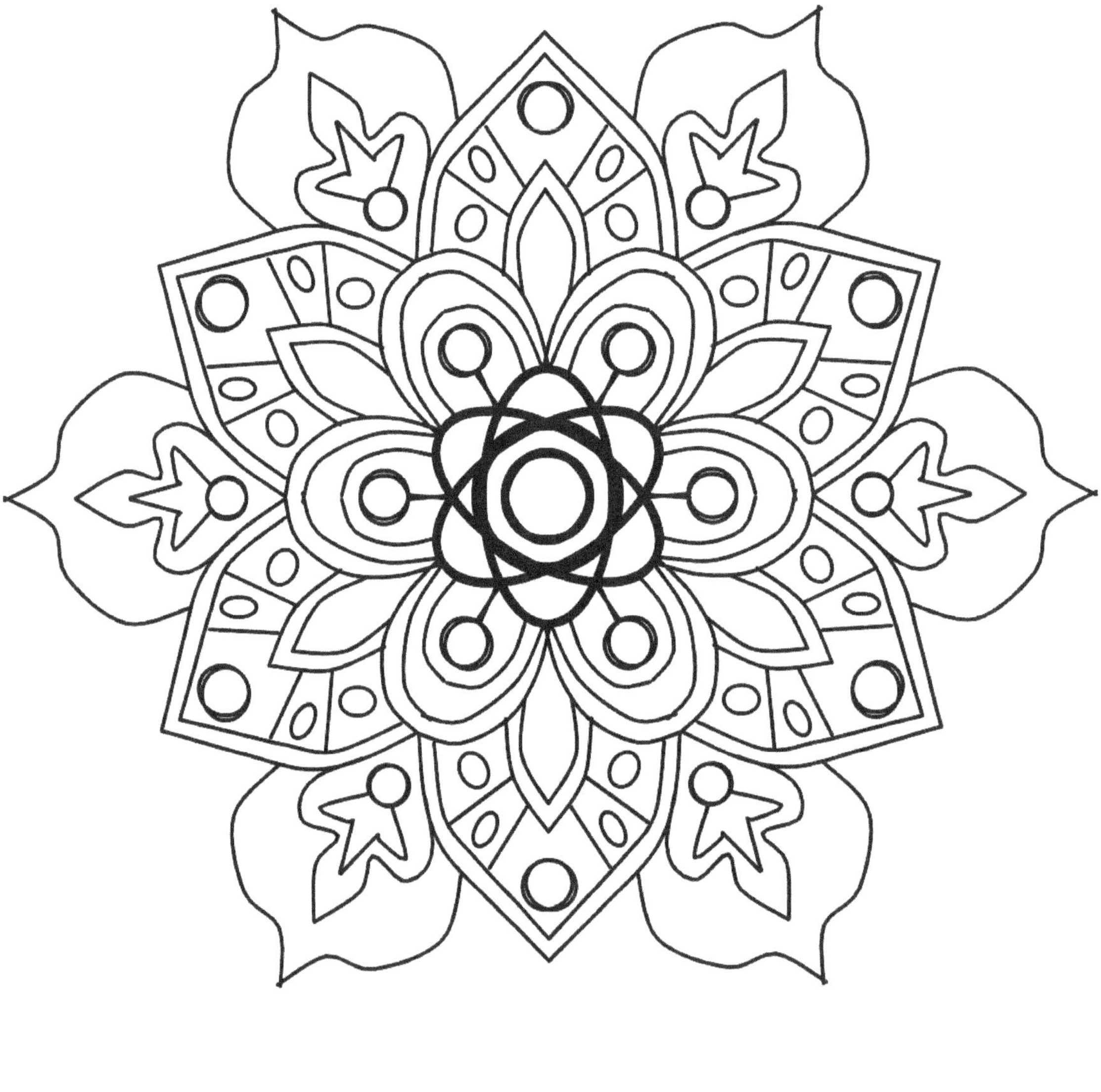

Day Twenty-four _______

5:00 _______________________

6:00 _______________________

7:00 _______________________

8:00 _______________________

9:00 _______________________

10:00 ______________________

11:00 ______________________

Noon _______________________

1:00 _______________________

2:00 _______________________

3:00 _______________________

4:00 _______________________

5:00 _______________________

6:00 _______________________

7:00 _______________________

8:00 _______________________

9:00 _______________________

10:00 ______________________

11:00 ______________________

Midnight ____________________

top priorities for today 🎯

____

____

____

____

Today's victories 🏆

What can you set on fire
with your fierceness?

____

____

____

____

____

____

The Stella Society Workout

Exercise	Set 1	Set 2	Set 3	Set 4	Set 5	notes

Time started: _____________ Time ended: ______________

Location: ____

Feelings before training: 🙂 😐 🙁 😜 😠 😨 😊 😎

Feelings after training 🙂 😐 🙁 😜 😠 😨 😊 😎

NUTRITION

Meal 1

time eaten: _________

Meal 2

time eaten: _________

Meal 3

time eaten: _________

Meal 4

time eaten: _________

Meal 5

time eaten: _________

Hydration

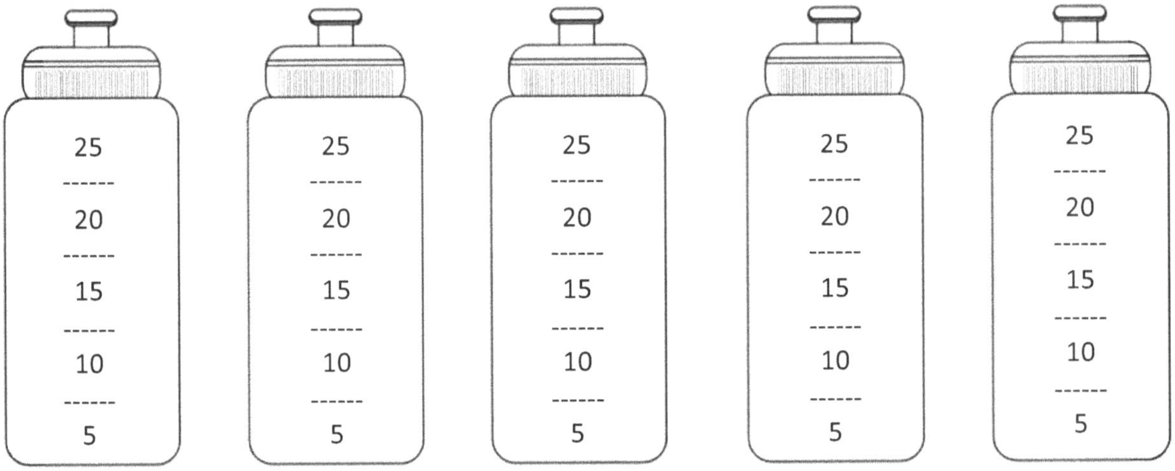

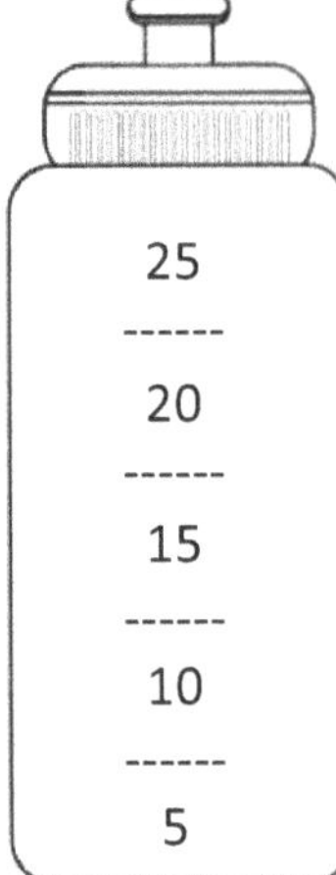

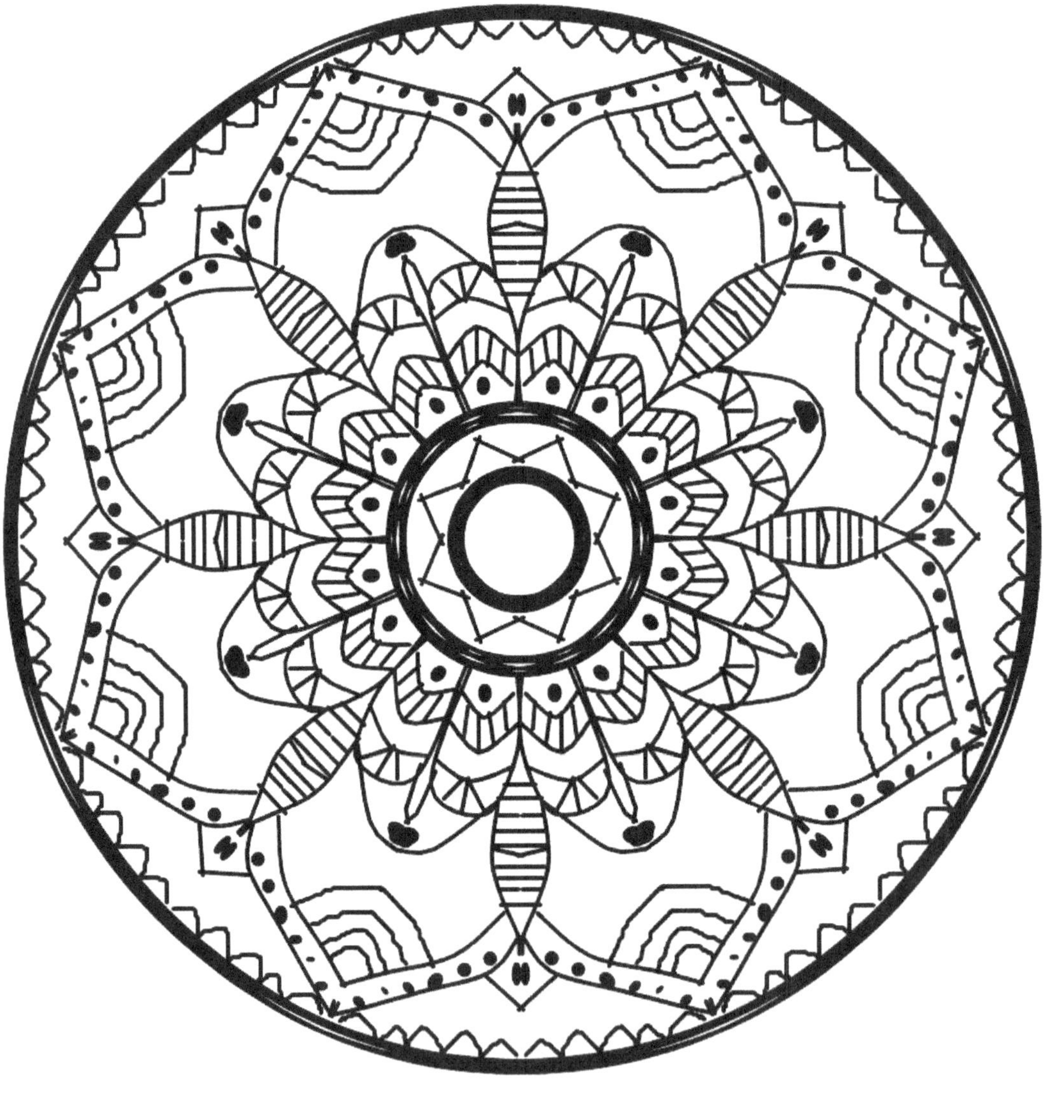

Day Twenty-five _______

5:00 _______________________

6:00 _______________________

7:00 _______________________

8:00 _______________________

9:00 _______________________

10:00 ______________________

11:00 ______________________

Noon _______________________

1:00 _______________________

2:00 _______________________

3:00 _______________________

4:00 _______________________

5:00 _______________________

6:00 _______________________

7:00 _______________________

8:00 _______________________

9:00 _______________________

10:00 ______________________

11:00 ______________________

Midnight ___________________

top priorities for today 🎯

____

____

____

____

Today's victories 🏆

Make it your mission to stay positive. Write your positive mission statement.

____

____

____

____

The Stella Society Workout

Exercise	Set 1	Set 2	Set 3	Set 4	Set 5	notes

Time started: _____________ Time ended: _______________

Location: ____

Feelings before training:

Feelings after training

NUTRITION

Meal 1
time eaten: _________

Meal 2
time eaten: _________

Meal 3
time eaten: _________

Meal 4
time eaten: _________

Meal 5
time eaten: _________

Hydration

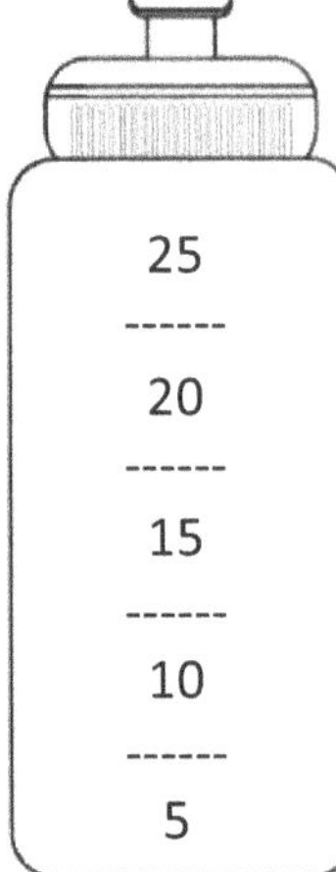

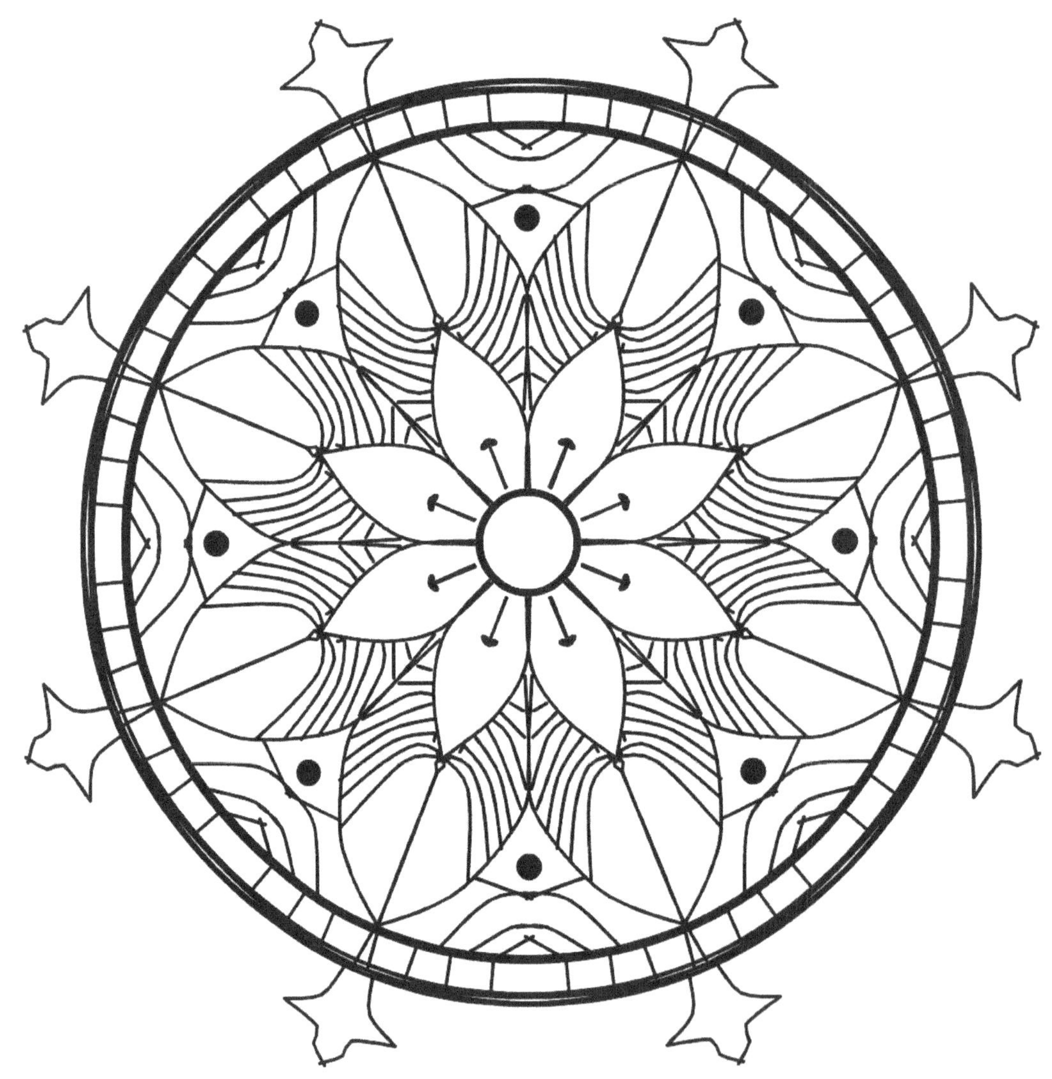

Day Twenty-six _______

5:00 _________________	

5:00 _____________________________
6:00 _____________________________
7:00 _____________________________
8:00 _____________________________
9:00 _____________________________
10:00 ____________________________
11:00 ____________________________
Noon _____________________________
1:00 _____________________________
2:00 _____________________________
3:00 _____________________________
4:00 _____________________________
5:00 _____________________________
6:00 _____________________________
7:00 _____________________________
8:00 _____________________________
9:00 _____________________________
10:00 ____________________________
11:00 ____________________________
Midnight _________________________

top priorities for today

____
____
____
____

Today's victories

What give you your inner energy?

____
____
____
____
____

The Stella Society Workout

Exercise	Set 1	Set 2	Set 3	Set 4	Set 5	notes

Time started: _____________ Time ended: _______________

Location: ____

Feelings before training: 🙂 😐 ☹️ 😝 😠 😔 😊 😎

Feelings after training 🙂 😐 ☹️ 😝 😠 😔 😊 😎

NUTRITION

Meal 1

time eaten: _________

Meal 2

time eaten: _________

Meal 3

time eaten: _________

Meal 4

time eaten: _________

Meal 5

time eaten: _________

Hydration

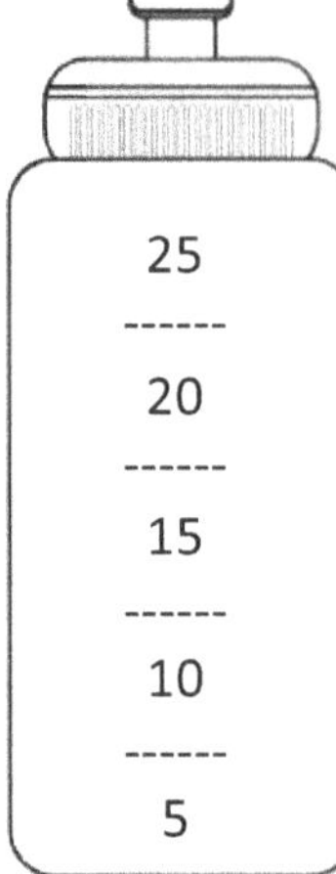

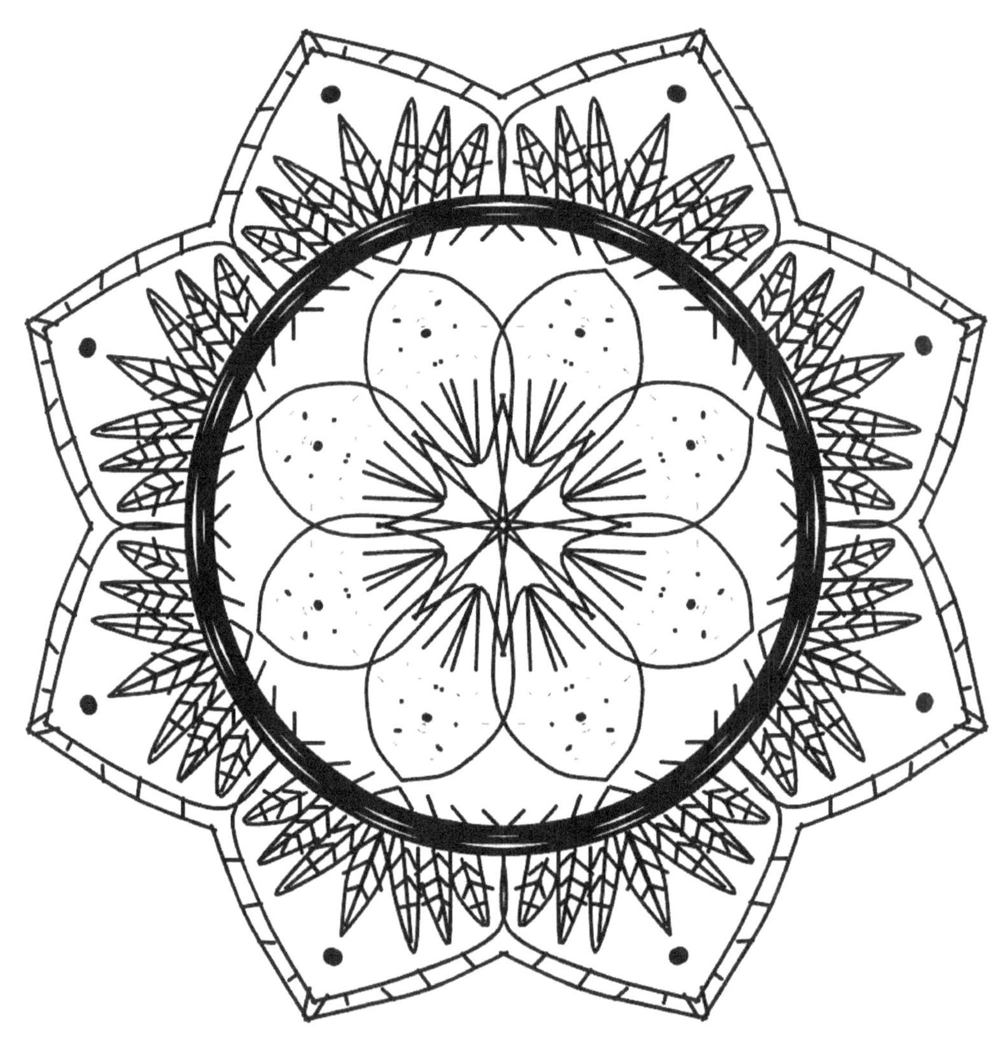

Day Twenty-seven _______

5:00 _______________________

6:00 _______________________

7:00 _______________________

8:00 _______________________

9:00 _______________________

10:00 ______________________

11:00 ______________________

Noon _______________________

1:00 _______________________

2:00 _______________________

3:00 _______________________

4:00 _______________________

5:00 _______________________

6:00 _______________________

7:00 _______________________

8:00 _______________________

9:00 _______________________

10:00 ______________________

11:00 ______________________

Midnight ____________________

top priorities for today 🎯

____

____

____

____

____

Today's victories 🏆

What have you stopped, but won't stop again?

____

____

____

____

____

The Stella Society Workout

Exercise	Set 1	Set 2	Set 3	Set 4	Set 5	notes

Time started: _____________ Time ended: _______________

Location: ____

Feelings before training: 🙂 😐 🙁 😜 😠 😕 😊 😎

Feelings after training 🙂 😐 🙁 😜 😠 😕 😊 😎

NUTRITION

Meal 1

time eaten: _________

Meal 2

time eaten: _________

Meal 3

time eaten: _________

Meal 4

time eaten: _________

Meal 5

time eaten: _________

Hydration

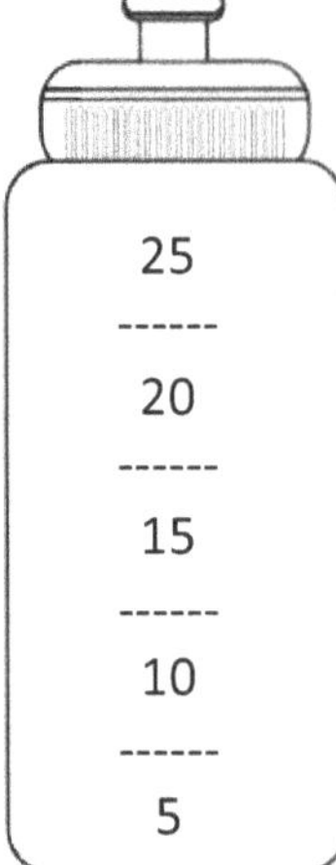
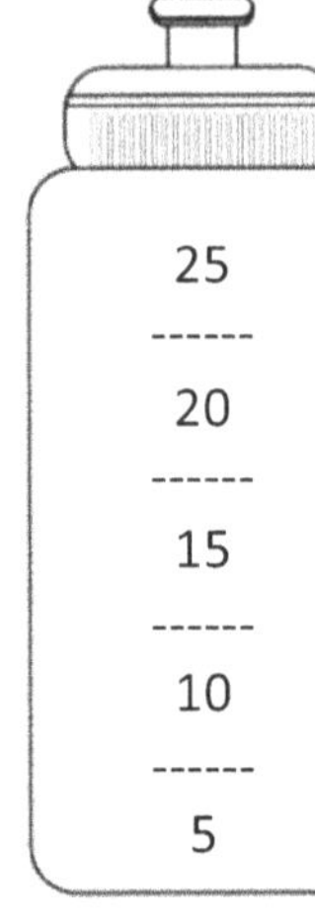
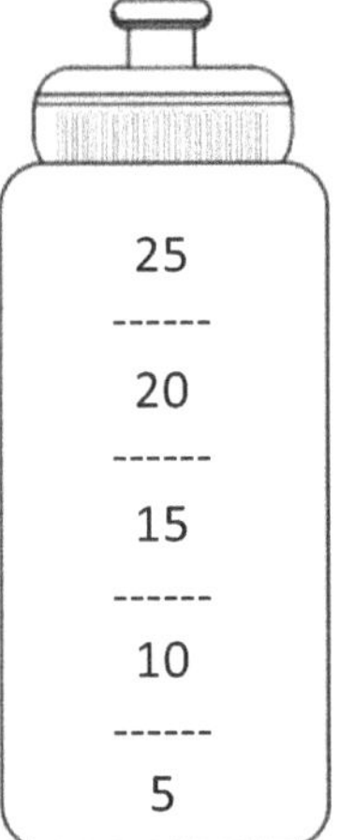
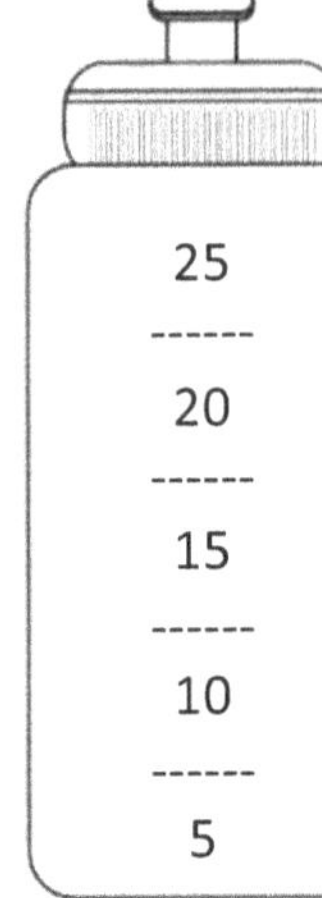
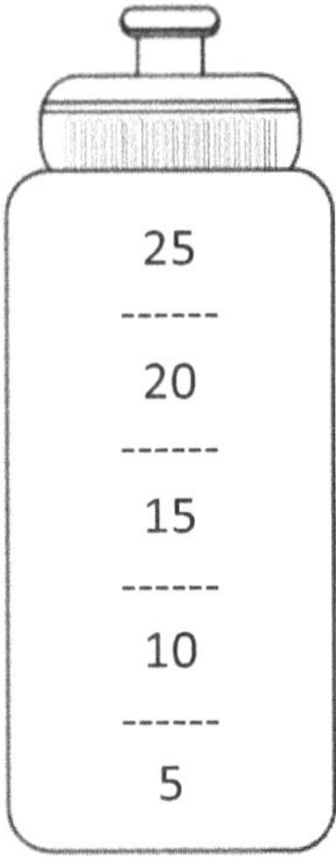

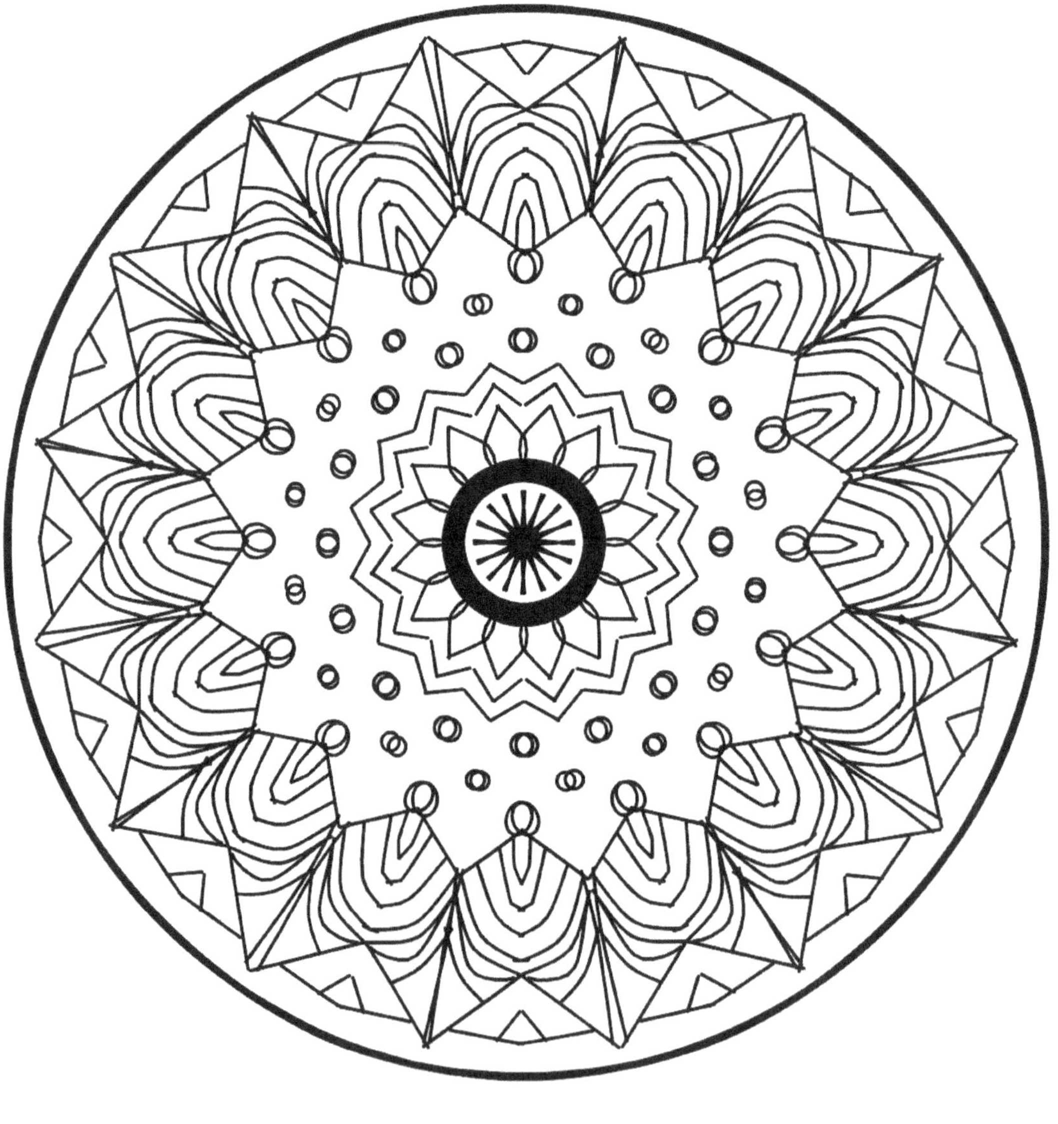

Day Twenty-eight _______

5:00 _______________	

5:00 ________________
6:00 ________________
7:00 ________________
8:00 ________________
9:00 ________________
10:00 ________________
11:00 ________________
Noon ________________
1:00 ________________
2:00 ________________
3:00 ________________
4:00 ________________
5:00 ________________
6:00 ________________
7:00 ________________
8:00 ________________
9:00 ________________
10:00 ________________
11:00 ________________
Midnight ________________

top priorities for today 🎯

____
____
____
____

Today's victories 🏆

How do identify with being
a unicorn?

____
____
____
____
____
____
____

The Stella Society Workout

Exercise	Set 1	Set 2	Set 3	Set 4	Set 5	notes

Time started: _______________ Time ended: _______________

Location: ____

Feelings before training:

Feelings after training

NUTRITION

Meal 1

time eaten: _________

Meal 2

time eaten: _________

Meal 3

time eaten: _________

Meal 4

time eaten: _________

Meal 5

time eaten: _________

Hydration

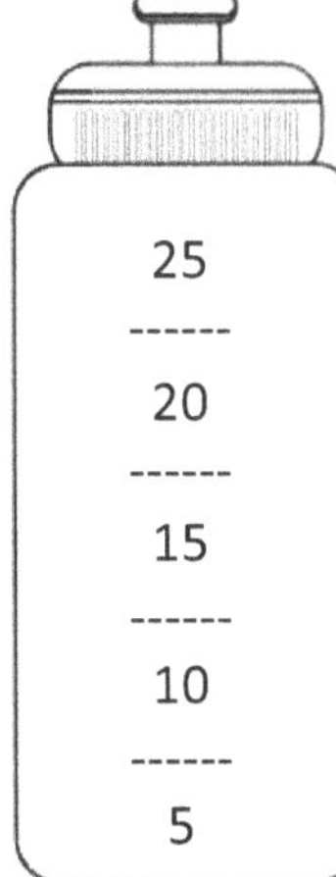

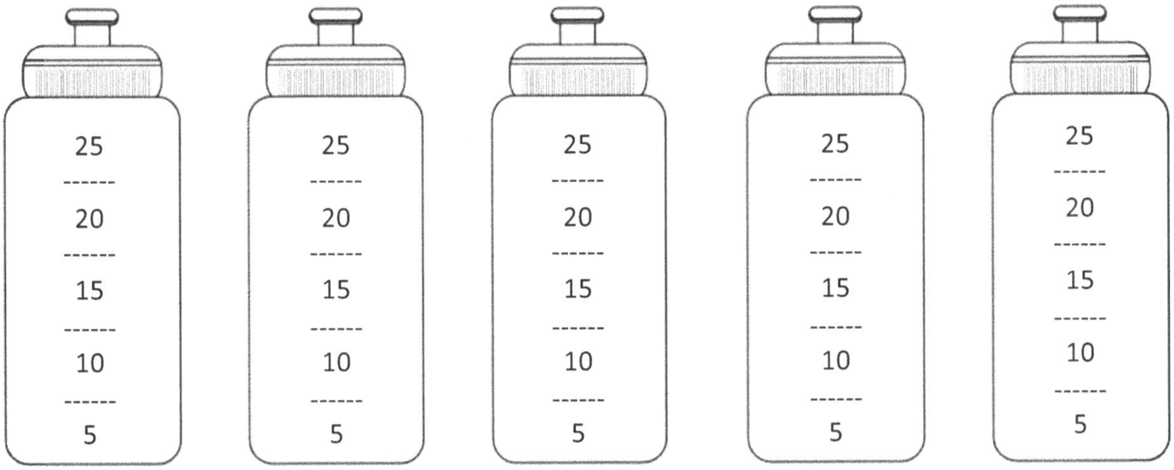

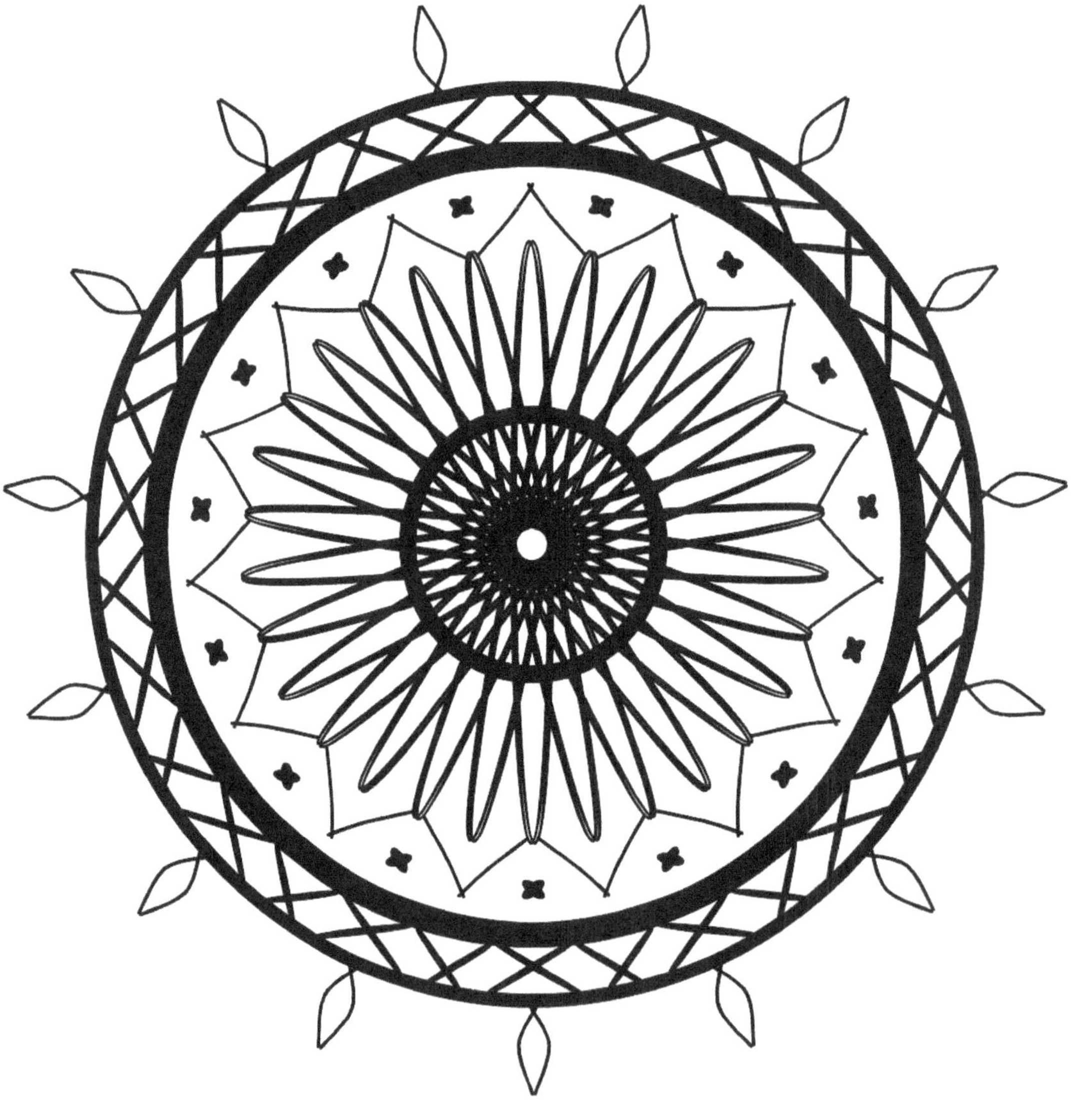

Day Twenty-nine ______

5:00 ______________________

6:00 ______________________

7:00 ______________________

8:00 ______________________

9:00 ______________________

10:00 _____________________

11:00 _____________________

Noon ______________________

1:00 ______________________

2:00 ______________________

3:00 ______________________

4:00 ______________________

5:00 ______________________

6:00 ______________________

7:00 ______________________

8:00 ______________________

9:00 ______________________

10:00 _____________________

11:00 _____________________

Midnight ___________________

top priorities for today

Today's victories

You have permission to be a savage. What do you do with it?

The Stella Society Workout

Exercise	Set 1	Set 2	Set 3	Set 4	Set 5	notes

Time started: _____________ Time ended: _______________

Location: ____

Feelings before training:

Feelings after training

NUTRITION

Meal 1

time eaten: _________

Meal 2

time eaten: _________

Meal 3

time eaten: _________

Meal 4

time eaten: _________

Meal 5

time eaten: _________

Hydration

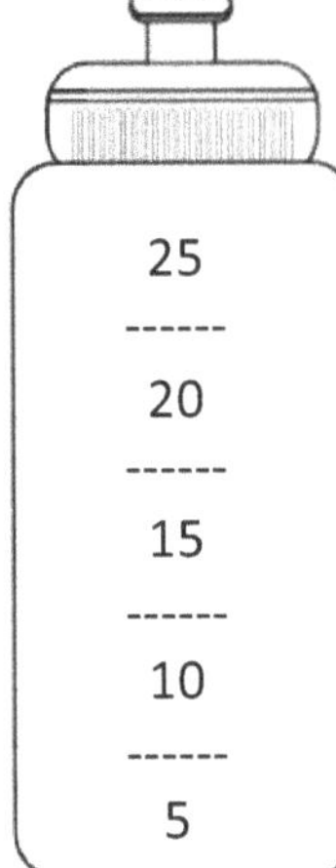

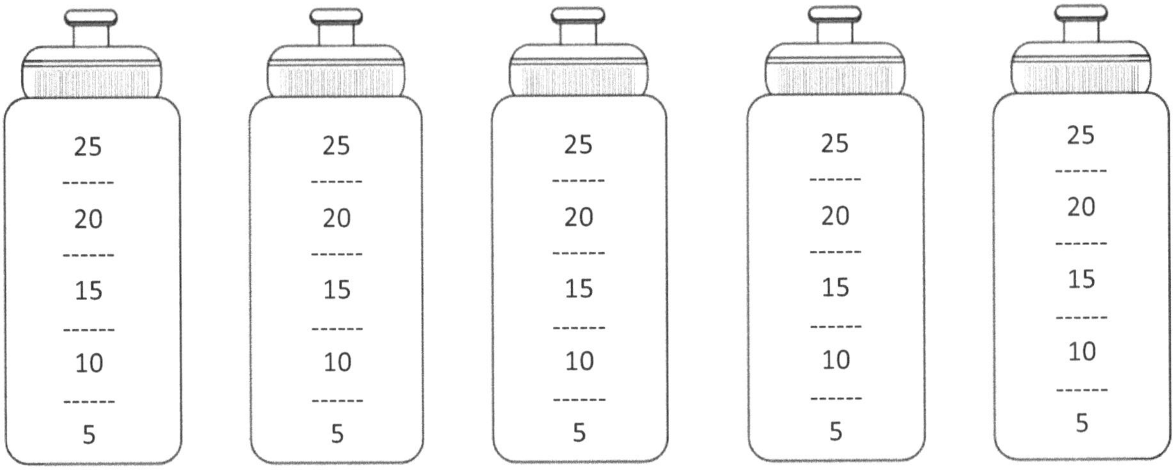

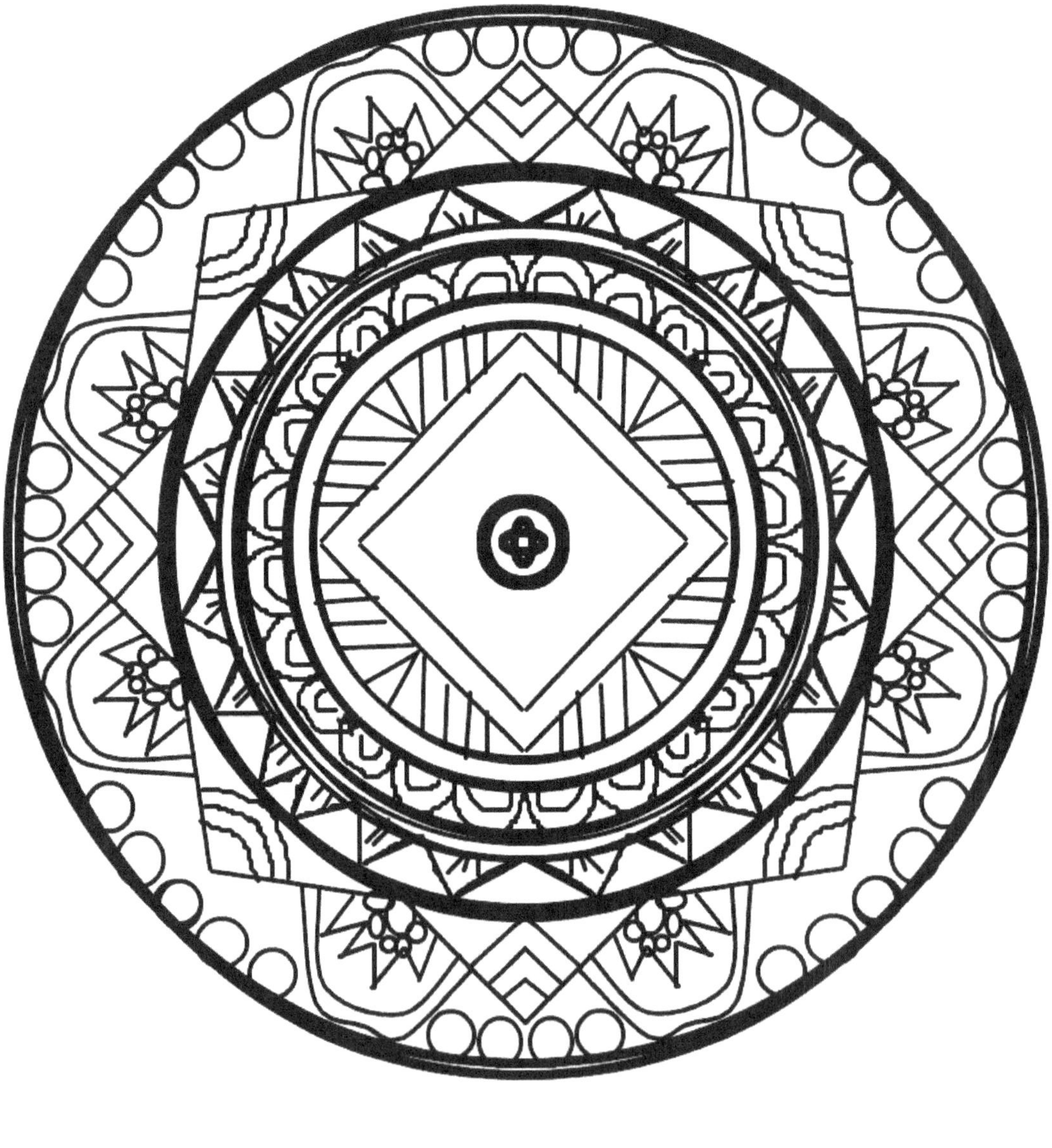

Measurements

DATE: ____________

Weight: _______

Neck _______

Shoulders _______

Chest _______

Bicep / upper arm left _________ right _______

Forearm left _________ right _______

Waist _______

Hips _______

Thighs left _________ right _______

Calf left _________ right _______

It's Not A Diet,
It's A Lifestyle Change

Day Thirty _______

5:00 _______________________

6:00 _______________________

7:00 _______________________

8:00 _______________________

9:00 _______________________

10:00 ______________________

11:00 ______________________

Noon _______________________

1:00 _______________________

2:00 _______________________

3:00 _______________________

4:00 _______________________

5:00 _______________________

6:00 _______________________

7:00 _______________________

8:00 _______________________

9:00 _______________________

10:00 ______________________

11:00 ______________________

Midnight ___________________

Today's victories

How can you be powerful and sensitive at the same time?

The Stella Society Workout

Exercise	Set 1	Set 2	Set 3	Set 4	Set 5	notes

Time started: _____________   Time ended: _____________

Location: ____

Feelings before training: 🙂 😐 🙁 😜 😠 😕 😊 😎

Feelings after training 🙂 😐 🙁 😜 😠 😕 😊 😎

NUTRITION

Meal 1

time eaten: _________

Meal 2

time eaten: _________

Meal 3

time eaten: _________

Meal 4

time eaten: _________

Meal 5

time eaten: _________

Hydration

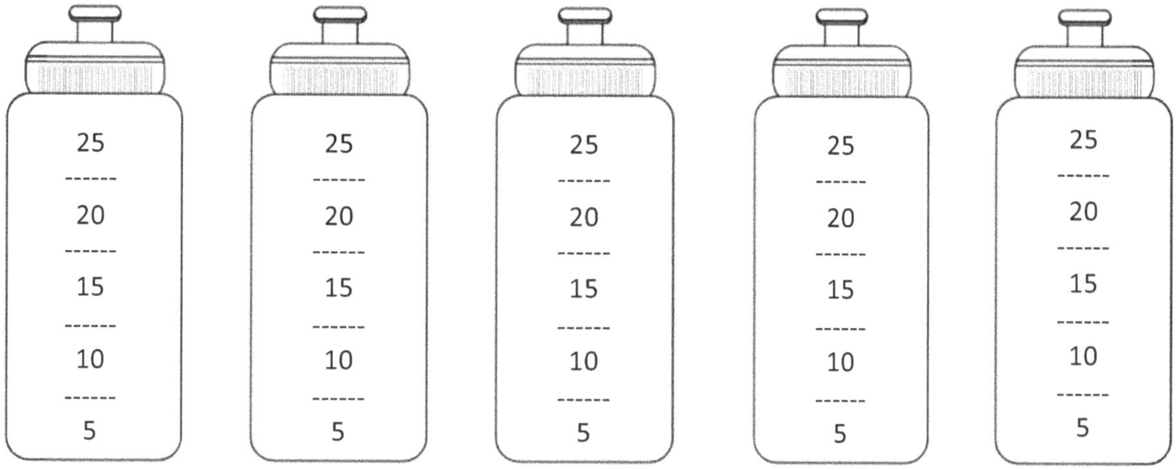

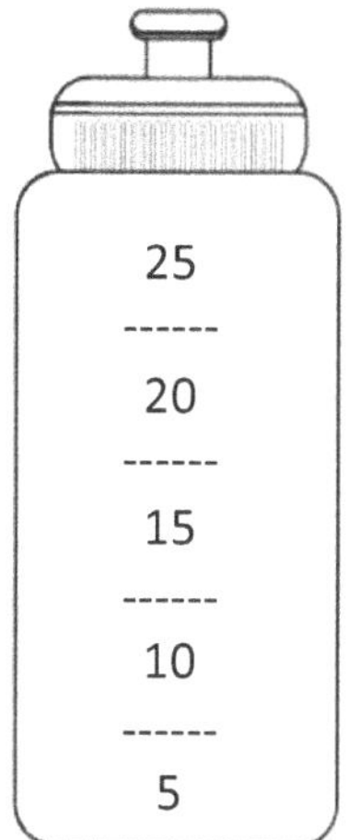 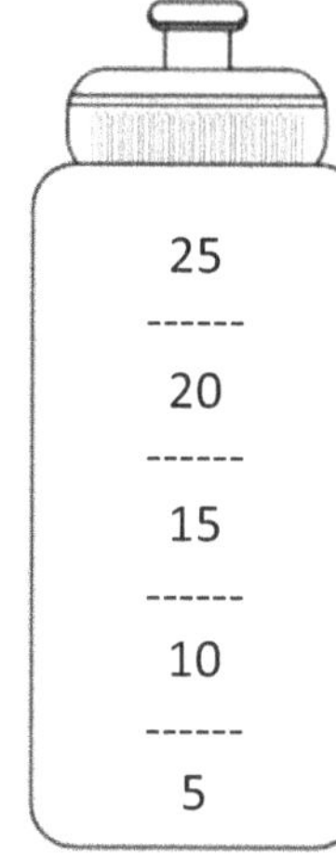 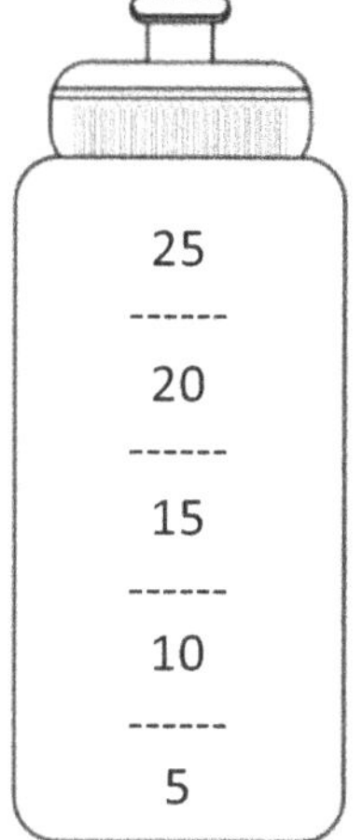

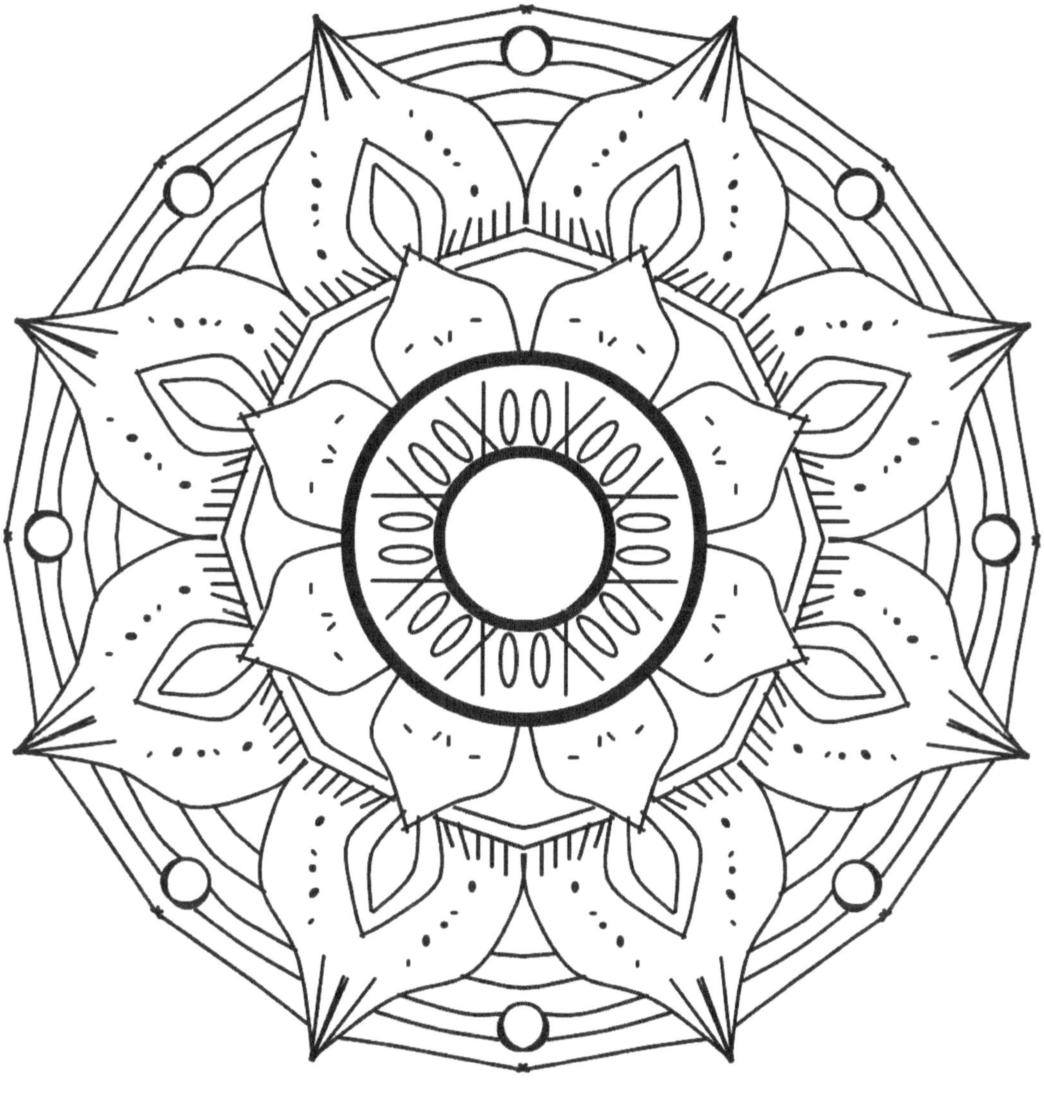

Day Thirty-one ______

5:00 ________________________

6:00 ________________________

7:00 ________________________

8:00 ________________________

9:00 ________________________

10:00 _______________________

11:00 _______________________

Noon _______________________

1:00 ________________________

2:00 ________________________

3:00 ________________________

4:00 ________________________

5:00 ________________________

6:00 ________________________

7:00 ________________________

8:00 ________________________

9:00 ________________________

10:00 _______________________

11:00 _______________________

Midnight ___________________

Is being forceful a bad thing?

The *Stella Society* Workout

Exercise	Set 1	Set 2	Set 3	Set 4	Set 5	notes

Time started: _____________ Time ended: _____________

Location: ____

Feelings before training:

Feelings after training

NUTRITION

Meal 1

time eaten: _________

Meal 2

time eaten: _________

Meal 3

time eaten: _________

Meal 4

time eaten: _________

Meal 5

time eaten: _________

Hydration

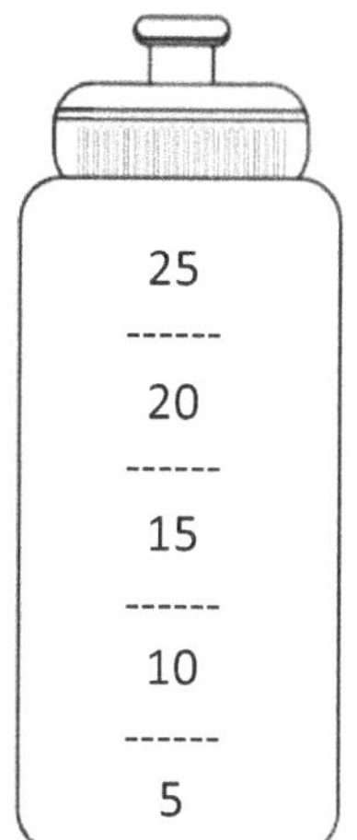
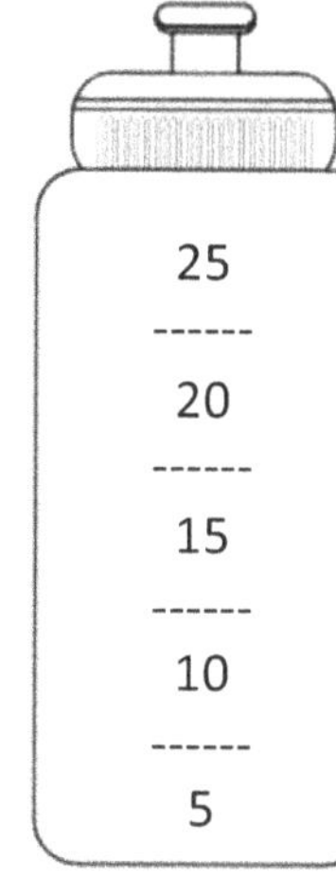
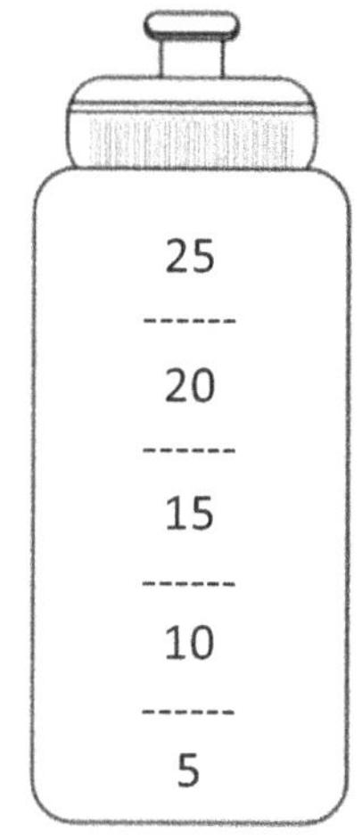
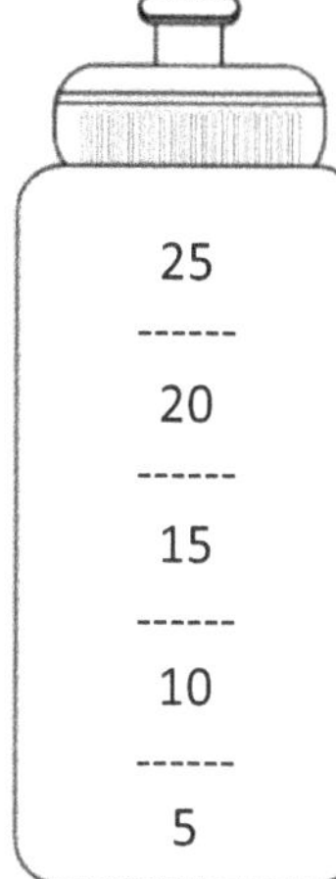
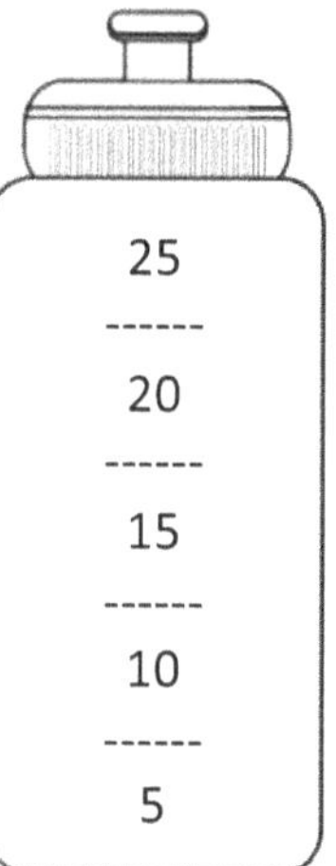

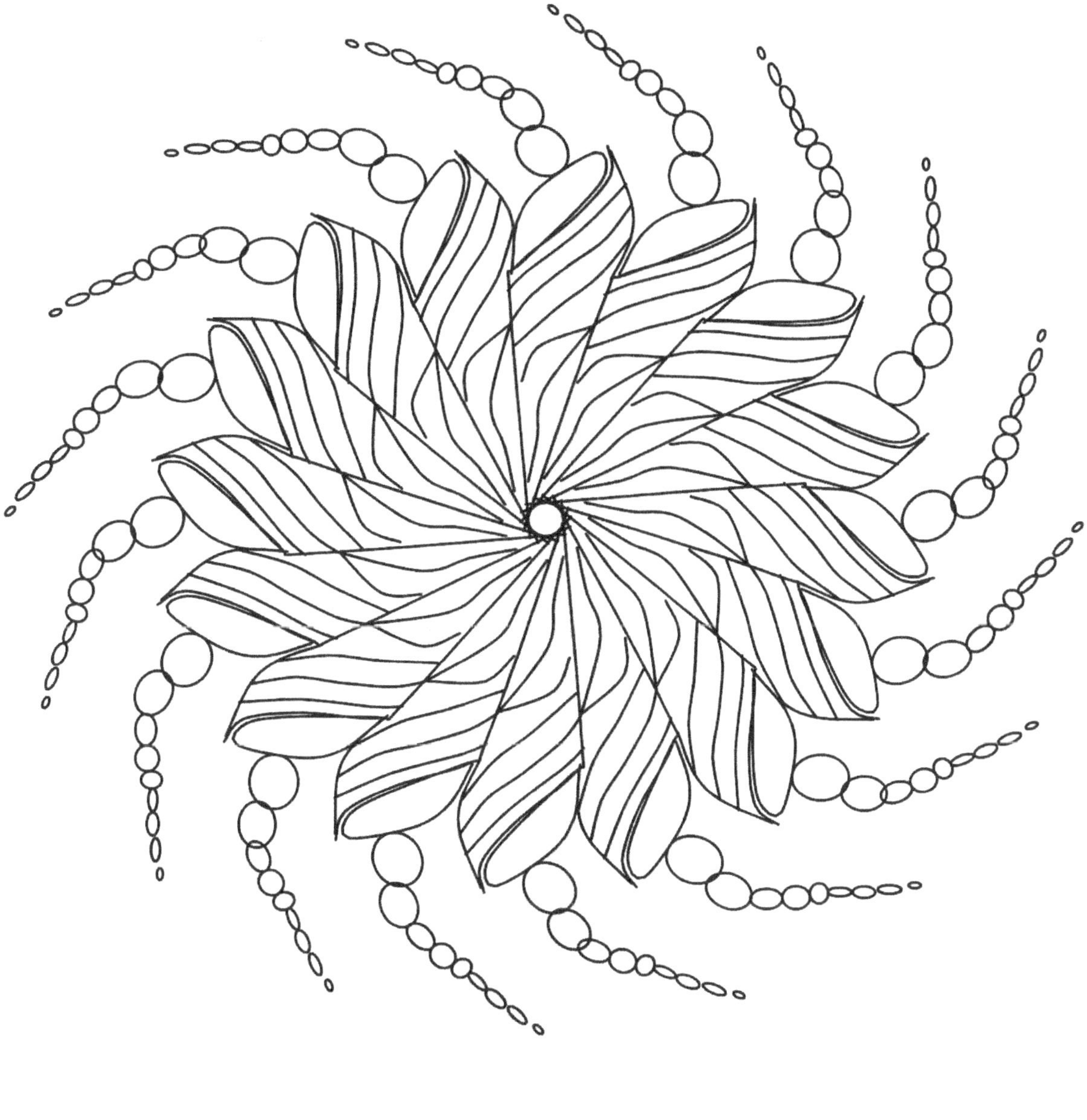

Day Thirty-two _______

5:00 _______________________

6:00 _______________________

7:00 _______________________

8:00 _______________________

9:00 _______________________

10:00 ______________________

11:00 ______________________

Noon _______________________

1:00 _______________________

2:00 _______________________

3:00 _______________________

4:00 _______________________

5:00 _______________________

6:00 _______________________

7:00 _______________________

8:00 _______________________

9:00 _______________________

10:00 ______________________

11:00 ______________________

Midnight ___________________

top priorities for today

____

____

____

____

____

Today's victories

What does it mean to be fervent?

____

____

____

____

____

____

The Workout

Stella Society

Exercise	Set 1	Set 2	Set 3	Set 4	Set 5	notes

Time started: _______________ Time ended: _______________

Location: ____

Feelings before training: 🙂 😐 🙁 😝 😠 🙁 😊 😎

Feelings after training 🙂 😐 🙁 😝 😠 🙁 😊 😎

NUTRITION

Meal 1
time eaten: __________

Meal 2
time eaten: __________

Meal 3
time eaten: __________

Meal 4
time eaten: __________

Meal 5
time eaten: __________

Hydration

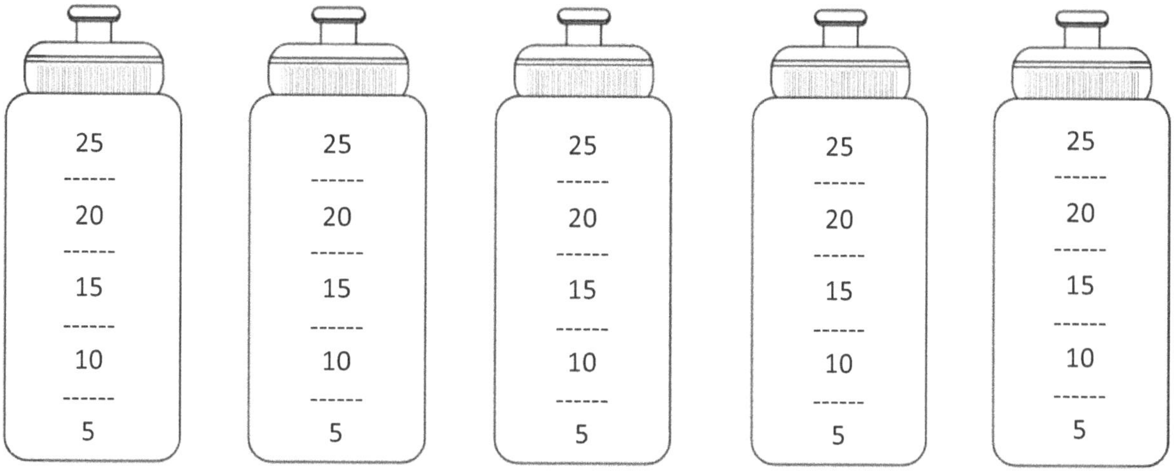

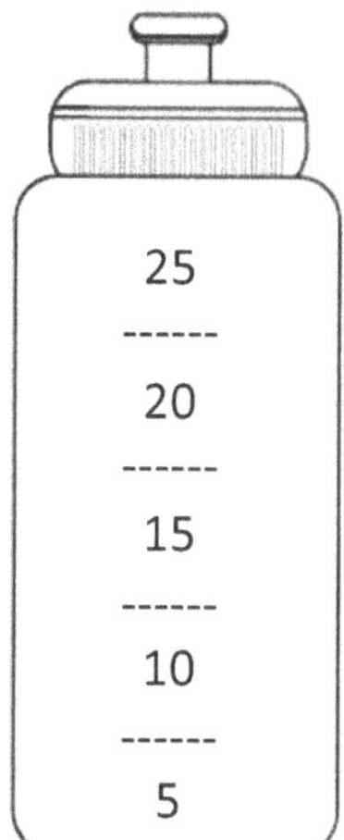
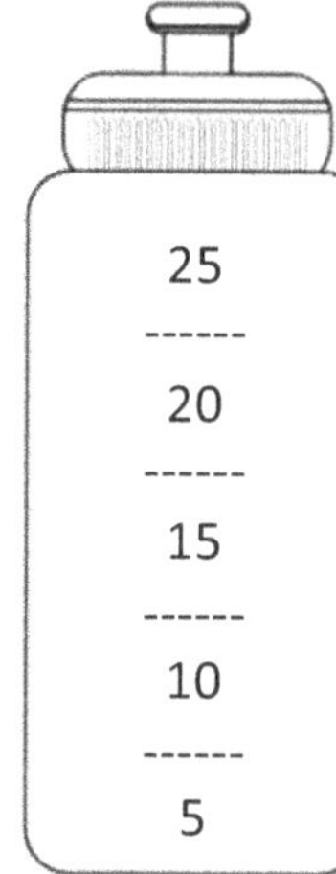
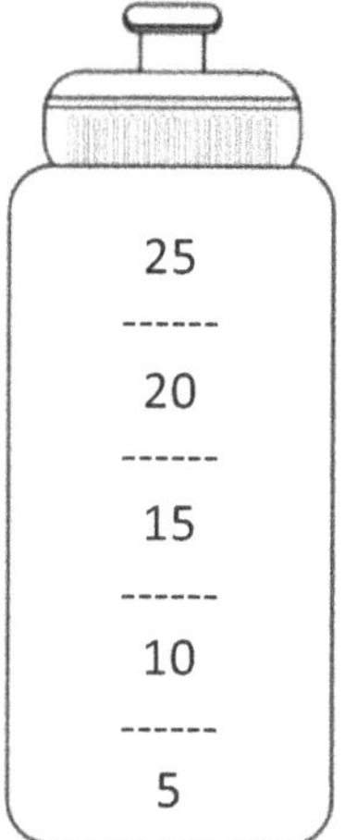
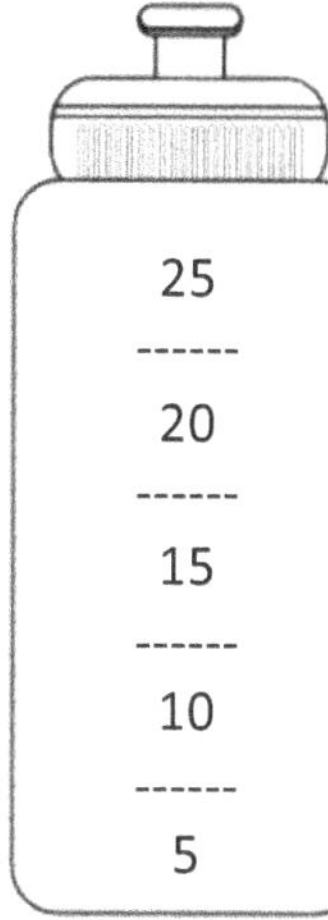

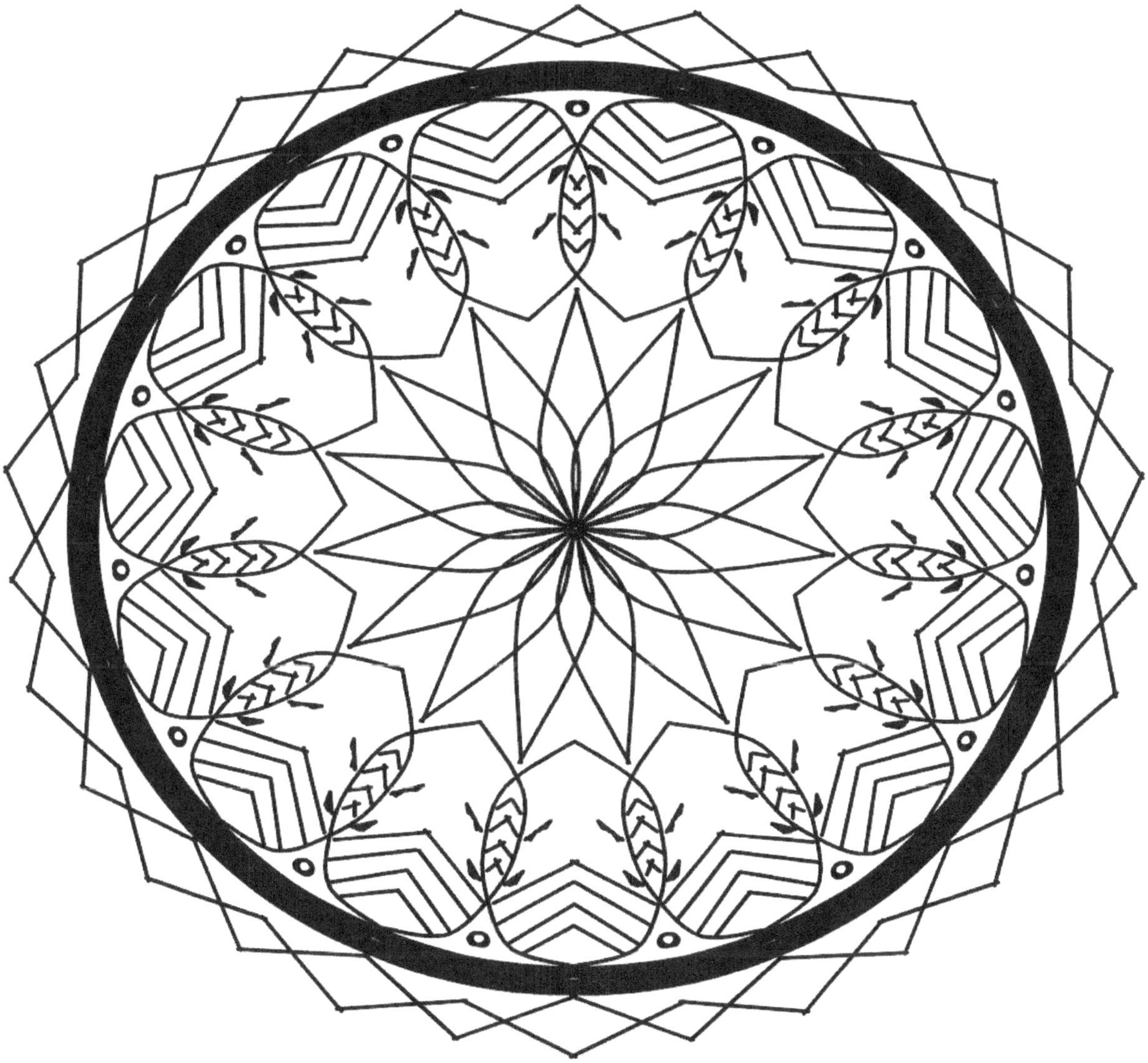

Day Thirty-three ______

5:00 ____________________	

5:00 ______________________

6:00 ______________________

7:00 ______________________

8:00 ______________________

9:00 ______________________

10:00 ____________________

11:00 ____________________

Noon _____________________

1:00 ______________________

2:00 ______________________

3:00 ______________________

4:00 ______________________

5:00 ______________________

6:00 ______________________

7:00 ______________________

8:00 ______________________

9:00 ______________________

10:00 ____________________

11:00 ____________________

Midnight _________________

top priorities for today

____

____

____

____

Today's victories

How are you glowing today?

____

____

____

____

____

____

The *Stella Society* Workout

Exercise	Set 1	Set 2	Set 3	Set 4	Set 5	notes

Time started: _____________ Time ended: _____________

Location: ____

Feelings before training: 🙂 😐 🙁 😜 😠 😟 😊 😎

Feelings after training 🙂 😐 🙁 😜 😠 😟 😊 😎

NUTRITION

Meal 1
time eaten: _________

Meal 2
time eaten: _________

Meal 3
time eaten: _________

Meal 4
time eaten: _________

Meal 5
time eaten: _________

Hydration

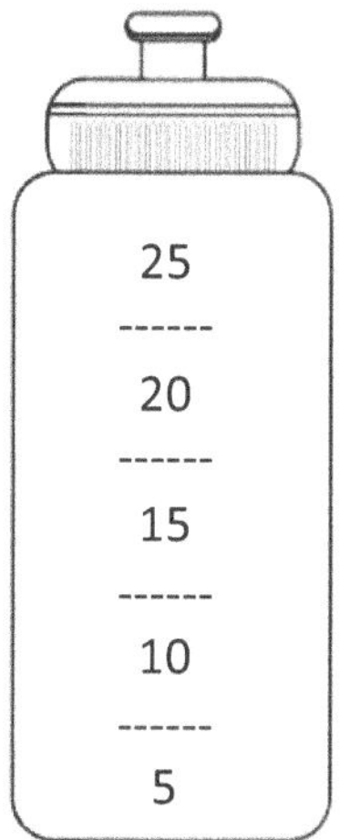

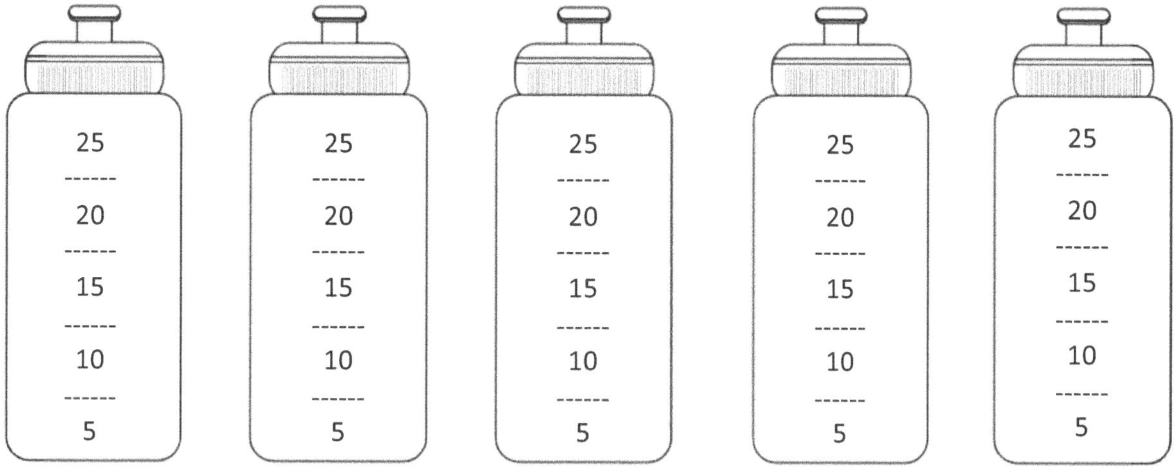

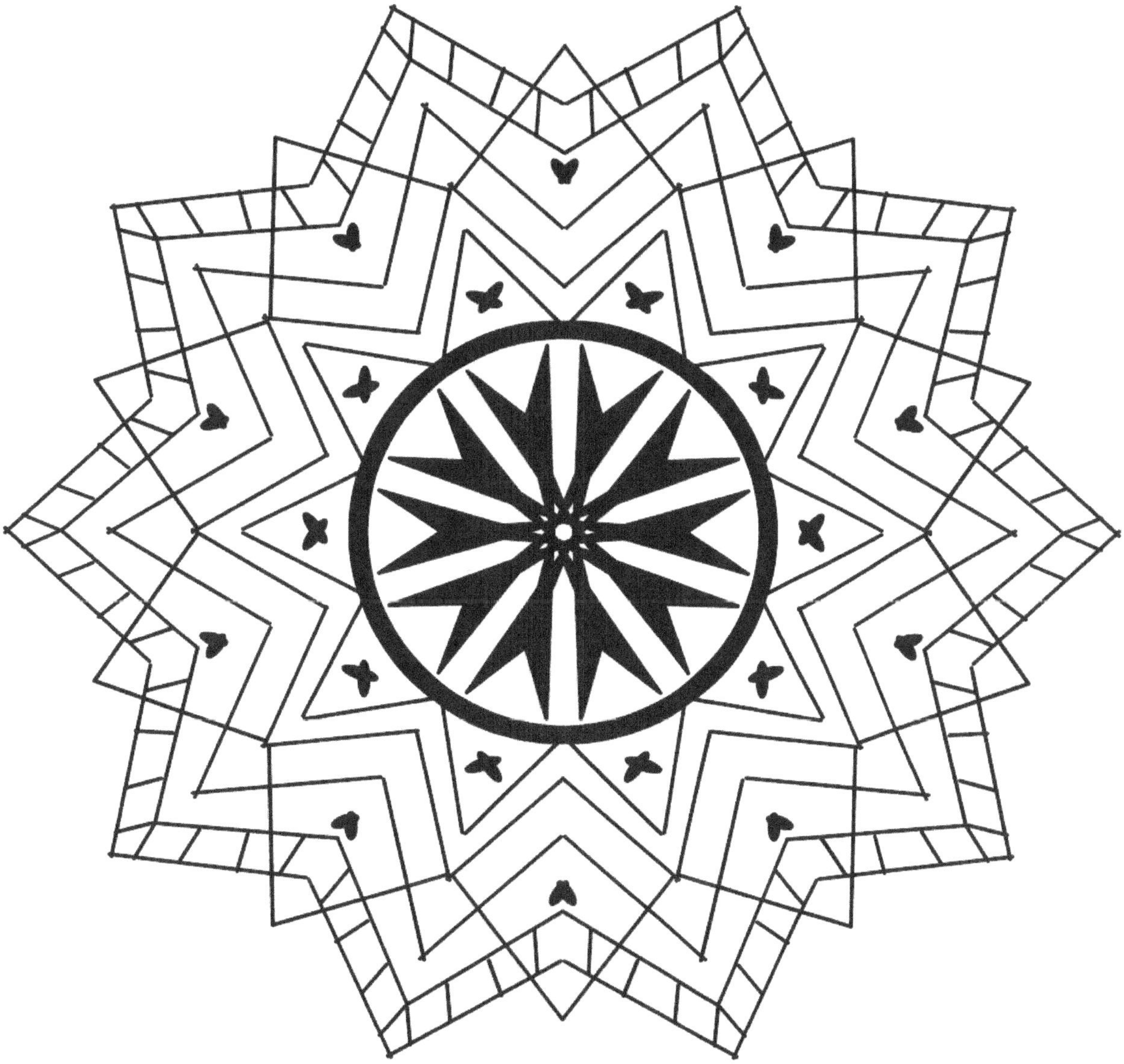

Day Thirty-four _______

Time	
5:00	_______________
6:00	_______________
7:00	_______________
8:00	_______________
9:00	_______________
10:00	_______________
11:00	_______________
Noon	_______________
1:00	_______________
2:00	_______________
3:00	_______________
4:00	_______________
5:00	_______________
6:00	_______________
7:00	_______________
8:00	_______________
9:00	_______________
10:00	_______________
11:00	_______________
Midnight	_______________

Today's victories

What are you dedicated to
do at this moment?

The Stella Society Workout

Exercise	Set 1	Set 2	Set 3	Set 4	Set 5	notes

Time started: _____________ Time ended: _____________

Location: ____

Feelings before training:        

Feelings after training

NUTRITION

Meal 1
time eaten: _________

Meal 2
time eaten: _________

Meal 3
time eaten: _________

Meal 4
time eaten: _________

Meal 5
time eaten: _________

Hydration

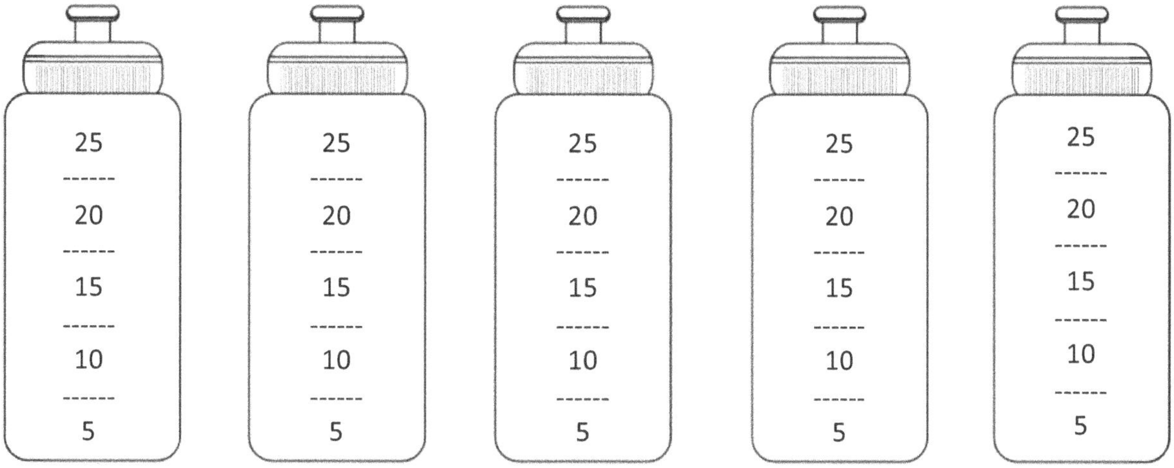

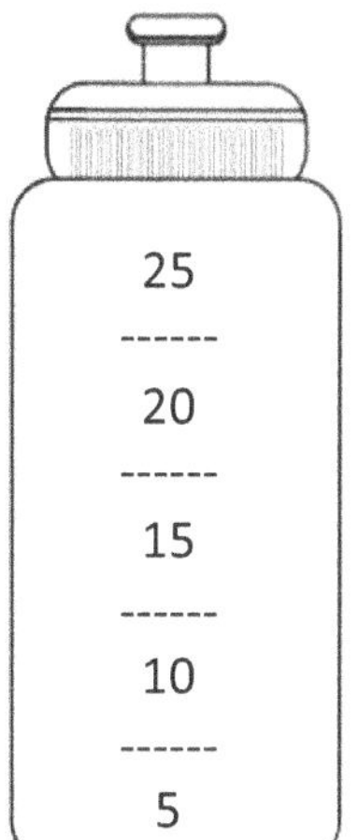
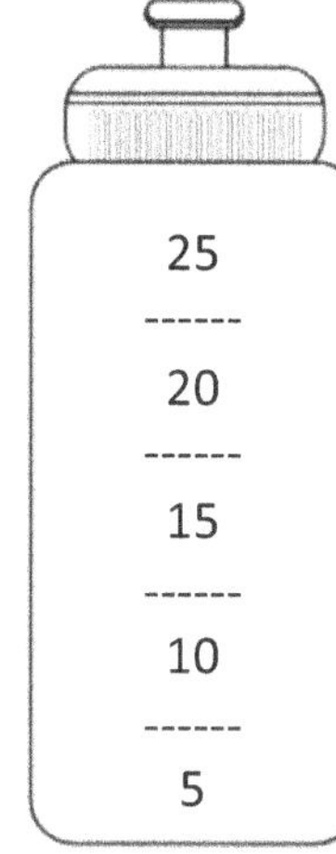
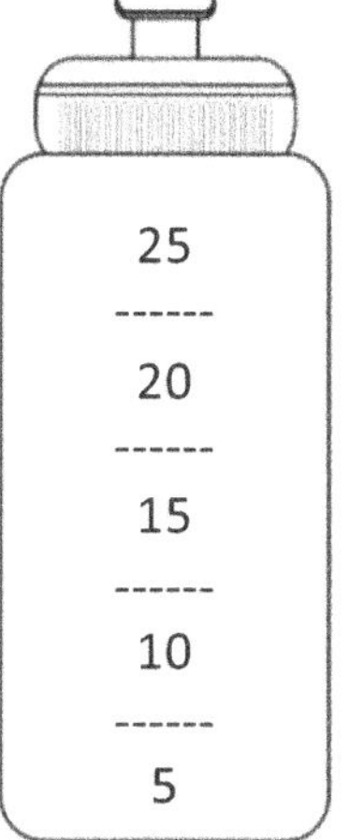
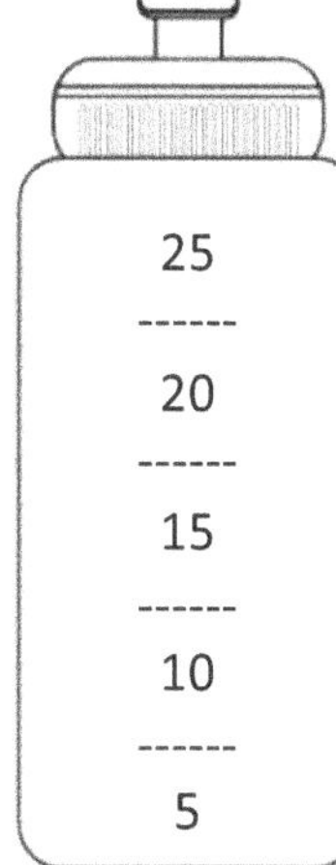
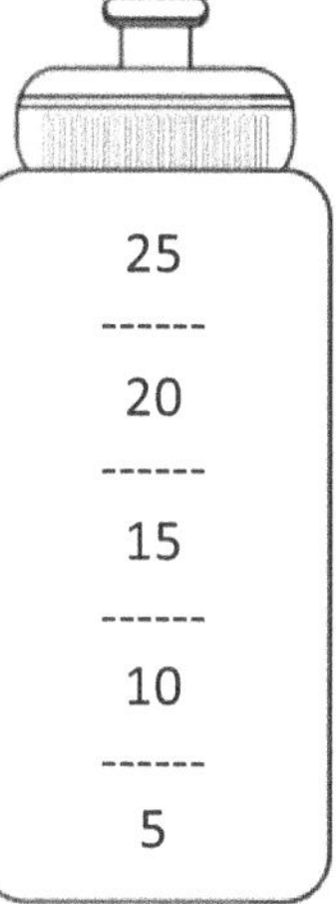

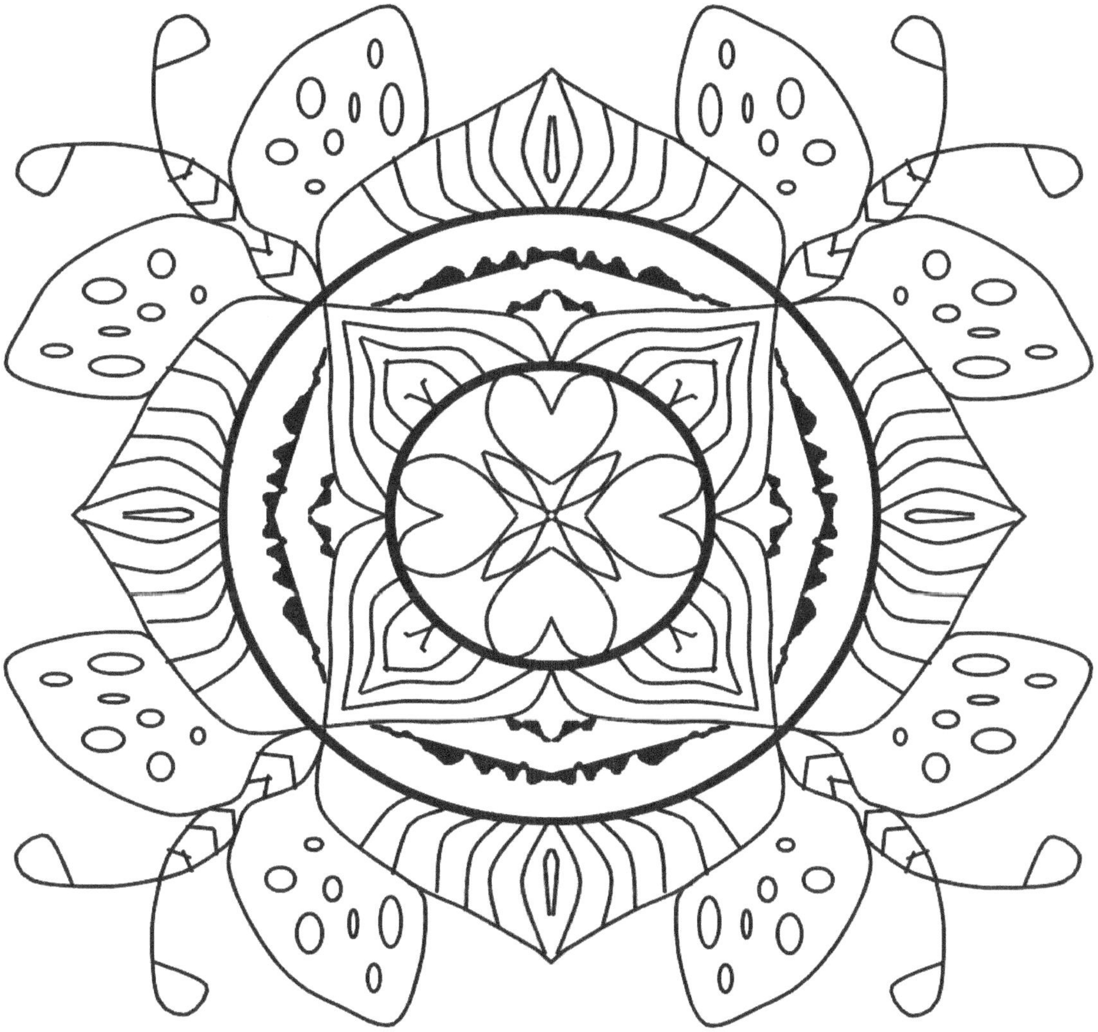

Day Thirty-five _______

5:00 _______________________

6:00 _______________________

7:00 _______________________

8:00 _______________________

9:00 _______________________

10:00 ______________________

11:00 ______________________

Noon _______________________

1:00 _______________________

2:00 _______________________

3:00 _______________________

4:00 _______________________

5:00 _______________________

6:00 _______________________

7:00 _______________________

8:00 _______________________

9:00 _______________________

10:00 ______________________

11:00 ______________________

Midnight ___________________

____

____

____

____

Today's victories

Who is more determined than you?

____

____

____

____

____

____

The Stella Society Workout

Exercise	Set 1	Set 2	Set 3	Set 4	Set 5	notes

Time started: _____________ Time ended: _____________

Location: ____

Feelings before training: 

Feelings after training

NUTRITION

Meal 1

time eaten: _________

Meal 2

time eaten: _________

Meal 3

time eaten: _________

Meal 4

time eaten: _________

Meal 5

time eaten: _________

Hydration

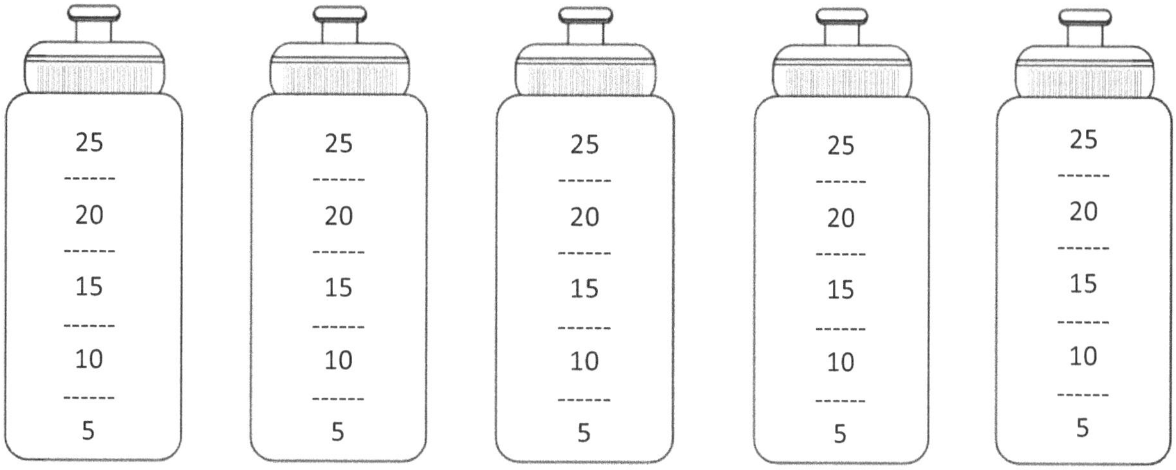

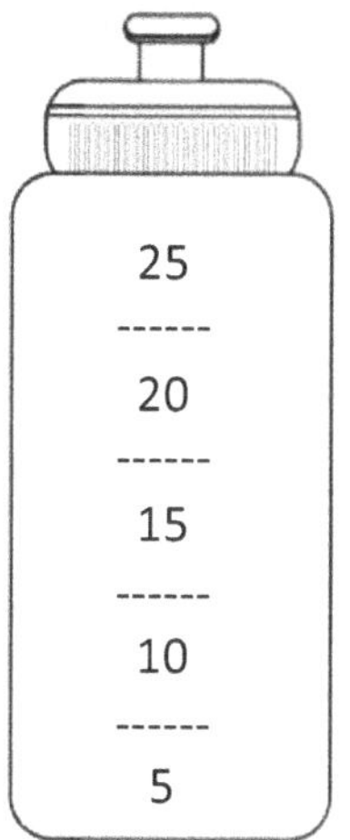
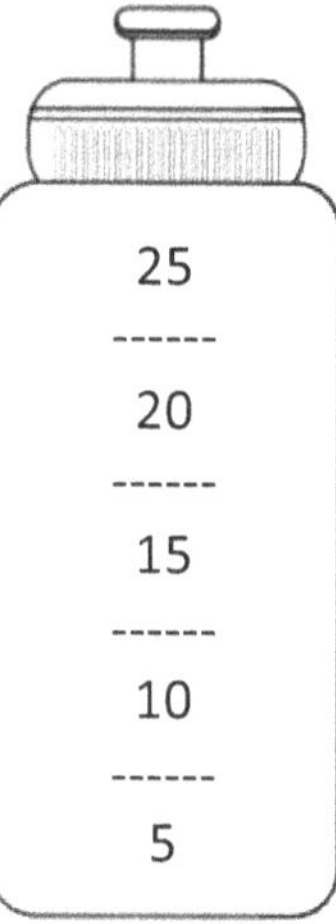

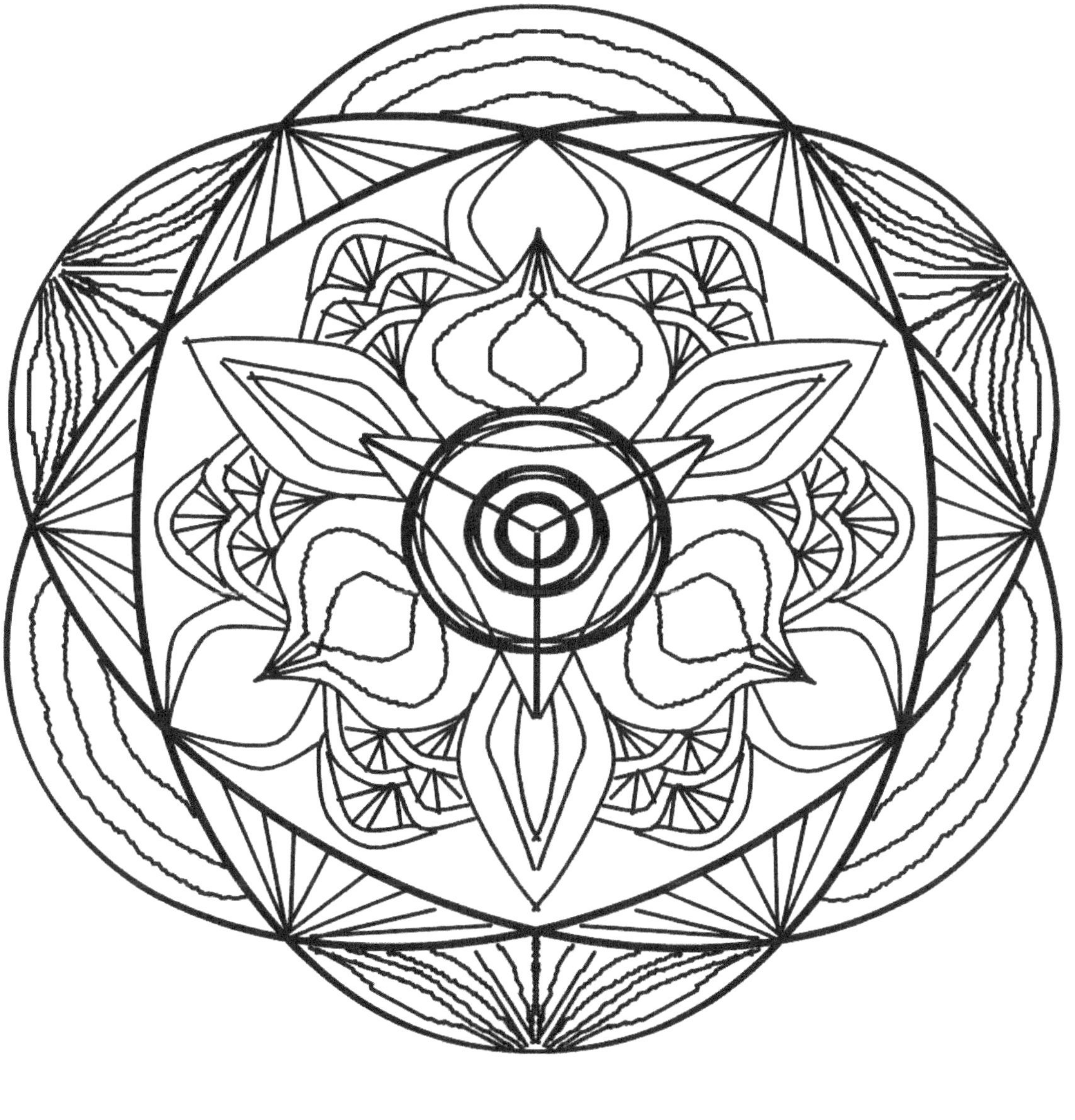

Day Thirty-six ______

top priorities for today

Today's victories

Who needs your acceptance
of change and why?

The Workout

Exercise	Set 1	Set 2	Set 3	Set 4	Set 5	notes

Time started: _______________ Time ended: _______________

Location: ____

Feelings before training:       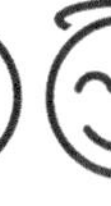 

Feelings after training

NUTRITION

Meal 1
time eaten: _________

Meal 2
time eaten: _________

Meal 3
time eaten: _________

Meal 4
time eaten: _________

Meal 5
time eaten: _________

Hydration

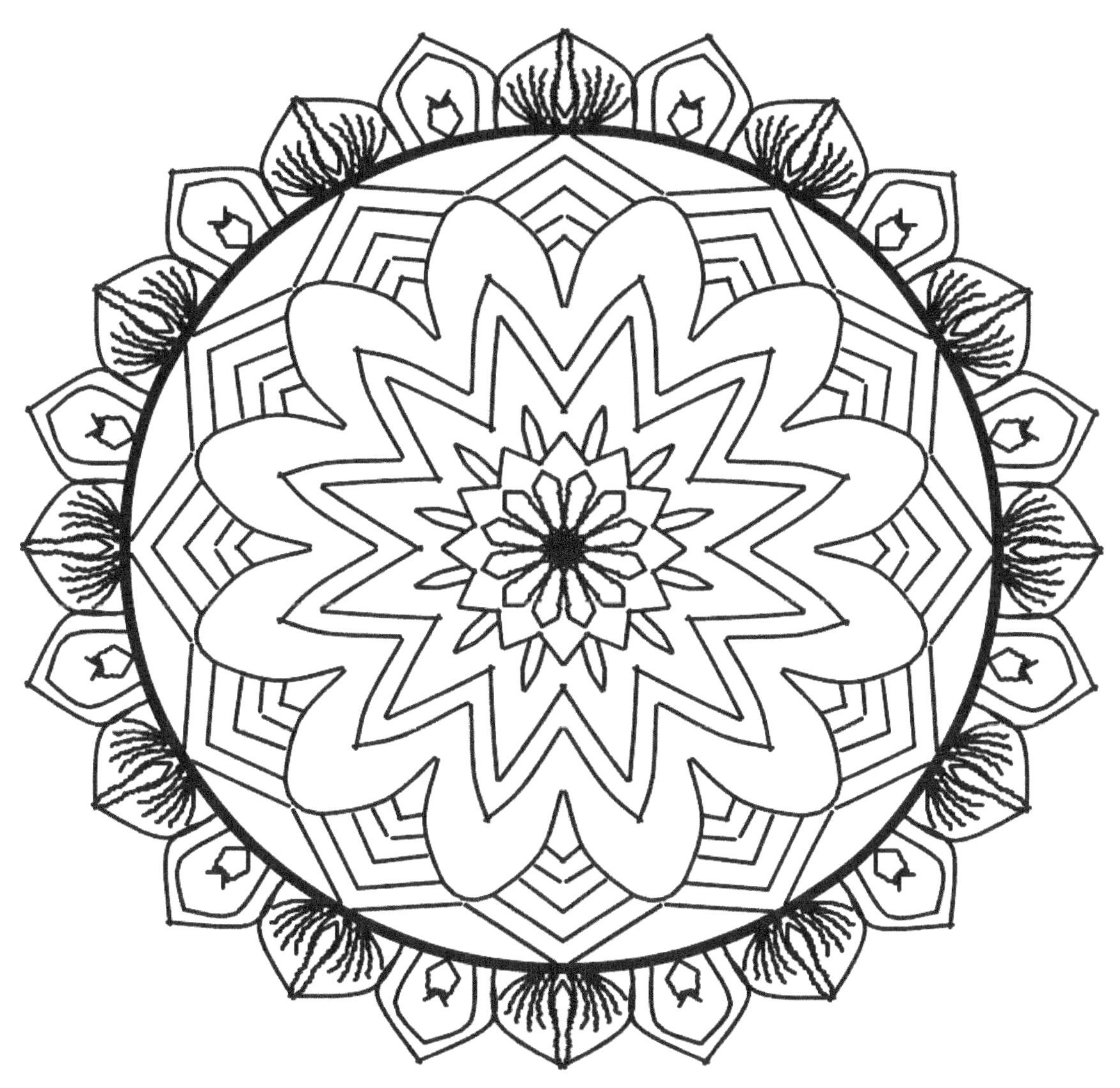

Day Thirty-seven _______

5:00 _______________________	top priorities for today
6:00 _______________________	

5:00 _______________________

6:00 _______________________

7:00 _______________________

8:00 _______________________

9:00 _______________________

10:00 _______________________

11:00 _______________________

Noon _______________________

1:00 _______________________

2:00 _______________________

3:00 _______________________

4:00 _______________________

5:00 _______________________

6:00 _______________________

7:00 _______________________

8:00 _______________________

9:00 _______________________

10:00 _______________________

11:00 _______________________

Midnight _______________________

top priorities for today

Today's victories

How will you be captivating?

The *Stella Society* Workout

Exercise	Set 1	Set 2	Set 3	Set 4	Set 5	notes

Time started: _____________ Time ended: _____________

Location: ____

Feelings before training: 🙂 😐 🙁 😝 😠 😒 😊 😎

Feelings after training 🙂 😐 🙁 😝 😠 😒 😊 😎

NUTRITION

Meal 1
time eaten: _________

Meal 2
time eaten: _________

Meal 3
time eaten: _________

Meal 4
time eaten: _________

Meal 5
time eaten: _________

Hydration

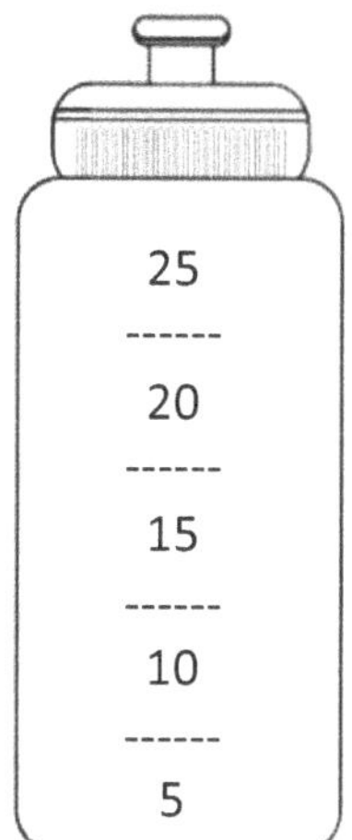

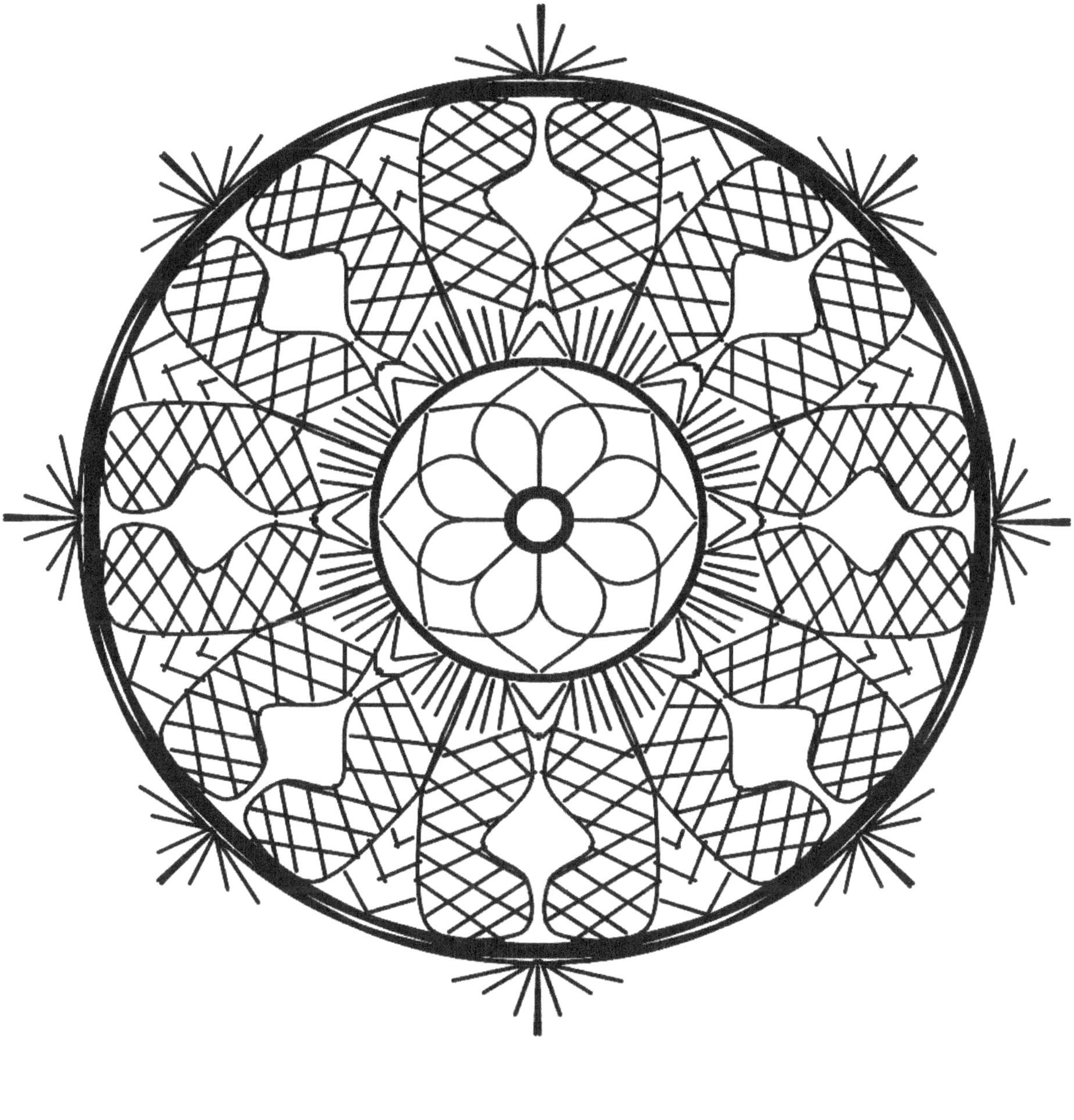

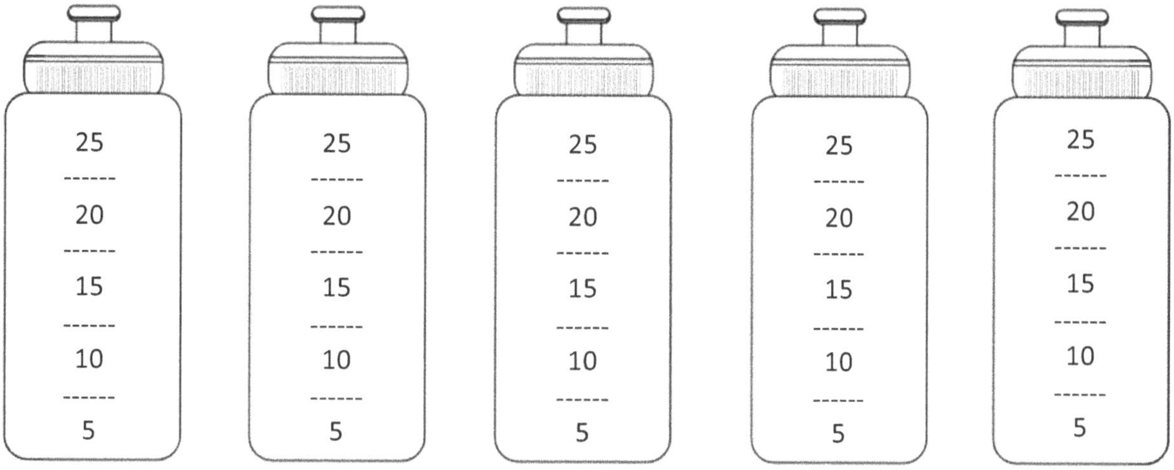

Day Thirty-eight _______

5:00 ______________________	

5:00 ______________________

6:00 ______________________

7:00 ______________________

8:00 ______________________

9:00 ______________________

10:00 _____________________

11:00 _____________________

Noon ______________________

1:00 ______________________

2:00 ______________________

3:00 ______________________

4:00 ______________________

5:00 ______________________

6:00 ______________________

7:00 ______________________

8:00 ______________________

9:00 ______________________

10:00 _____________________

11:00 _____________________

Midnight __________________

top priorities for today

____

____

____

____

____

Today's victories 🏆

What does it mean to be alluring?

____

____

____

____

____

____

____

The Stella Society Workout

Exercise	Set 1	Set 2	Set 3	Set 4	Set 5	notes

Time started: _______________   Time ended: _______________

Location: ____

Feelings before training:        

Feelings after training

NUTRITION

Meal 1

time eaten: _________

Meal 2

time eaten: _________

Meal 3

time eaten: _________

Meal 4

time eaten: _________

Meal 5

time eaten: _________

Hydration

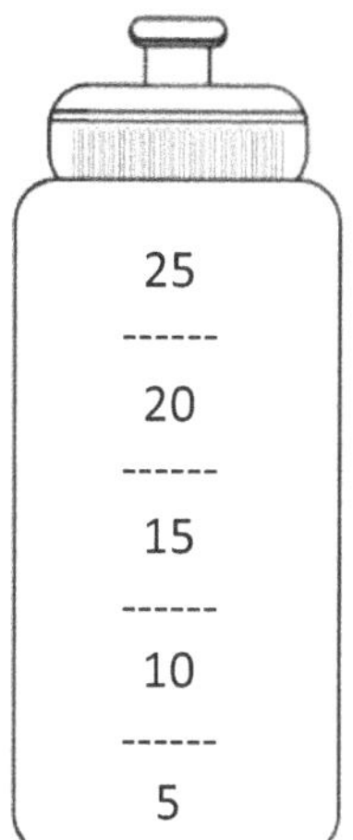
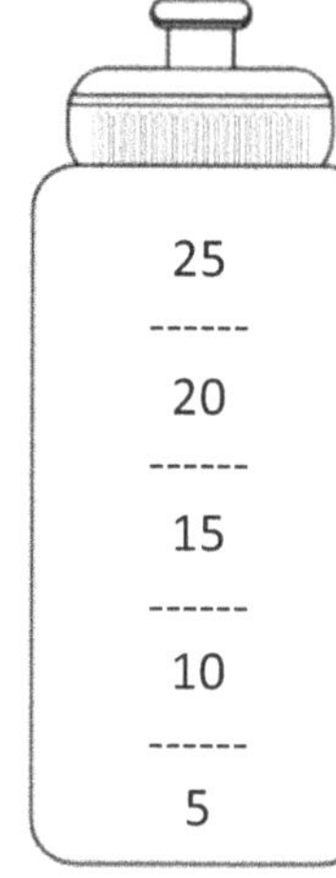
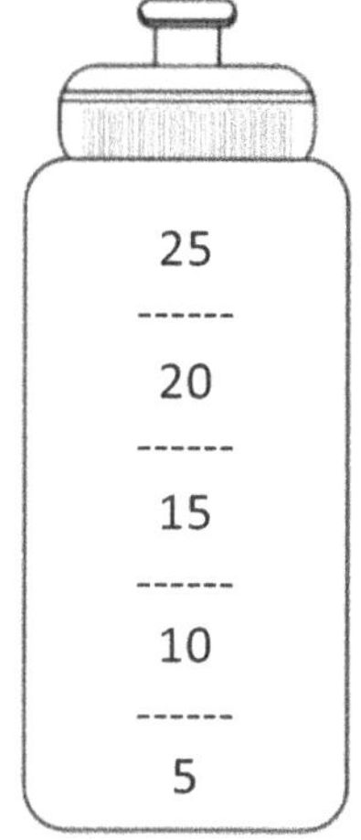
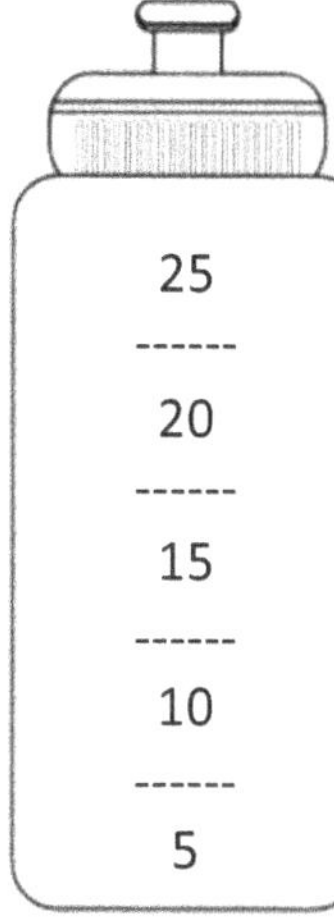
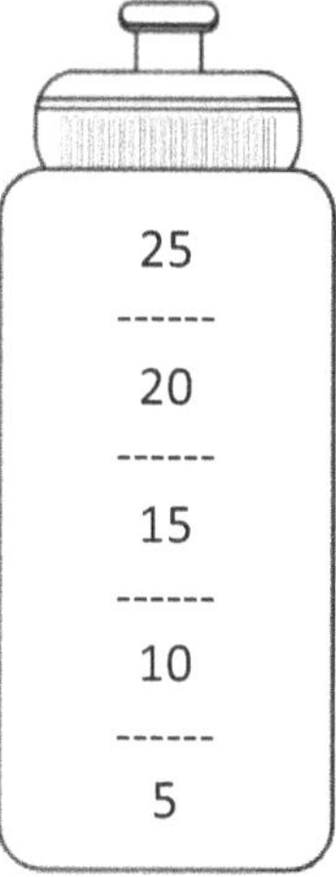

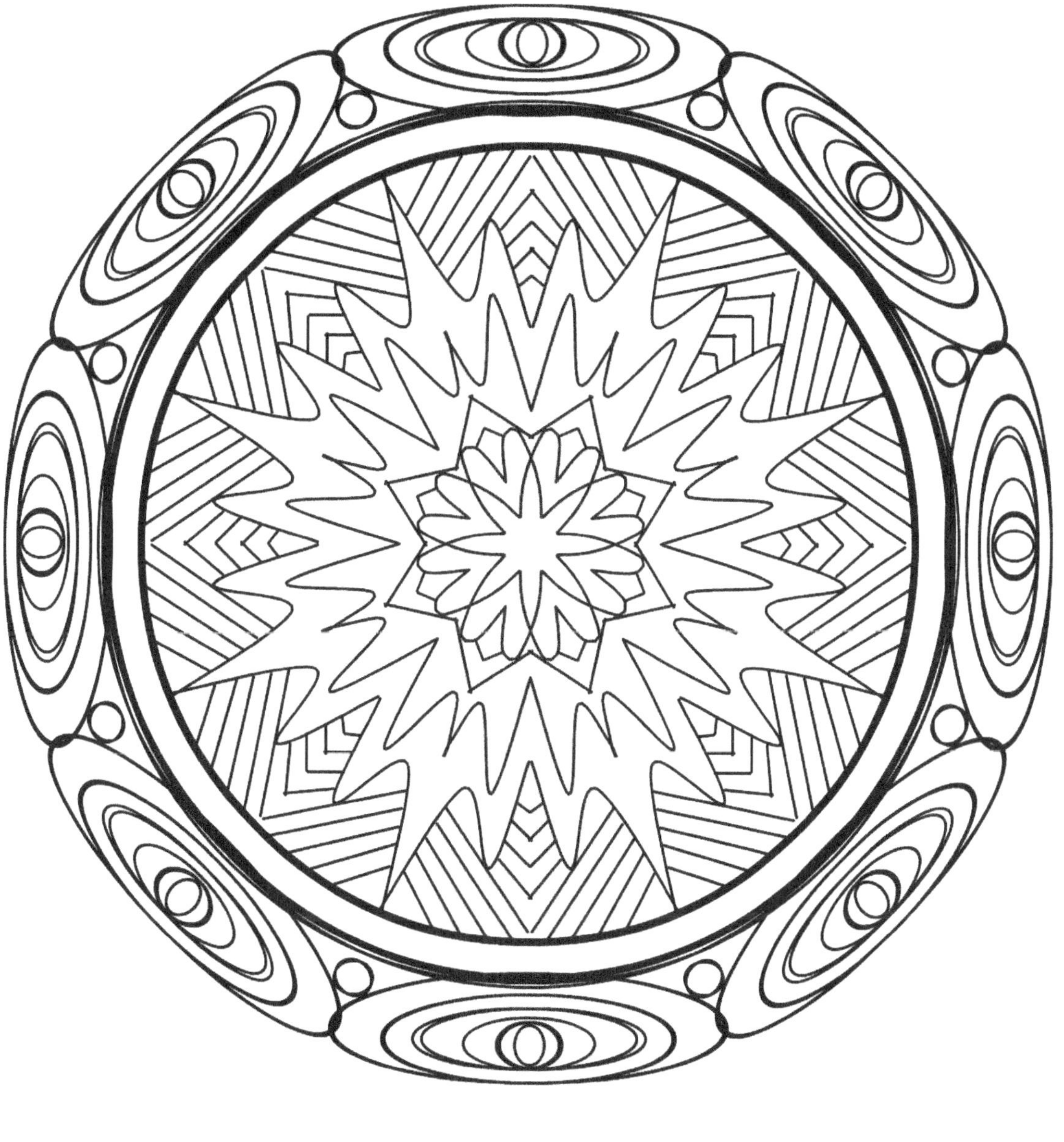

Day Thirty-nine _______

5:00 _______________________

6:00 _______________________

7:00 _______________________

8:00 _______________________

9:00 _______________________

10:00 ______________________

11:00 ______________________

Noon _______________________

1:00 _______________________

2:00 _______________________

3:00 _______________________

4:00 _______________________

5:00 _______________________

6:00 _______________________

7:00 _______________________

8:00 _______________________

9:00 _______________________

10:00 ______________________

11:00 ______________________

Midnight ____________________

top priorities for today

____

____

____

____

Today's victories

How will you be the best
version of you?

____

____

____

____

____

____

____

The Stella Society Workout

Exercise	Set 1	Set 2	Set 3	Set 4	Set 5	notes

Time started: _______________ Time ended: _______________

Location: ____

Feelings before training:

Feelings after training

NUTRITION

Meal 1
time eaten: _________

Meal 2
time eaten: _________

Meal 3
time eaten: _________

Meal 4
time eaten: _________

Meal 5
time eaten: _________

Hydration

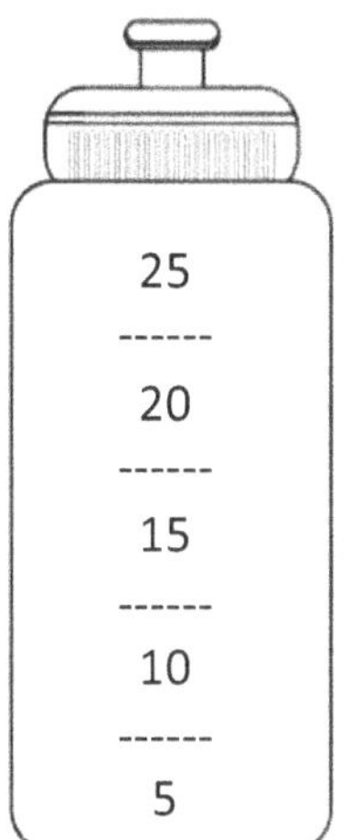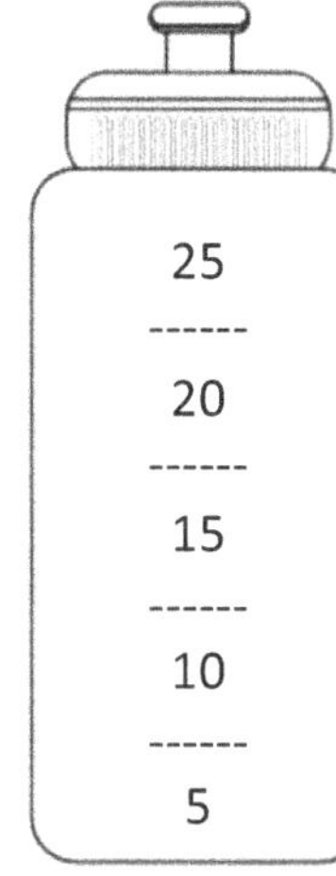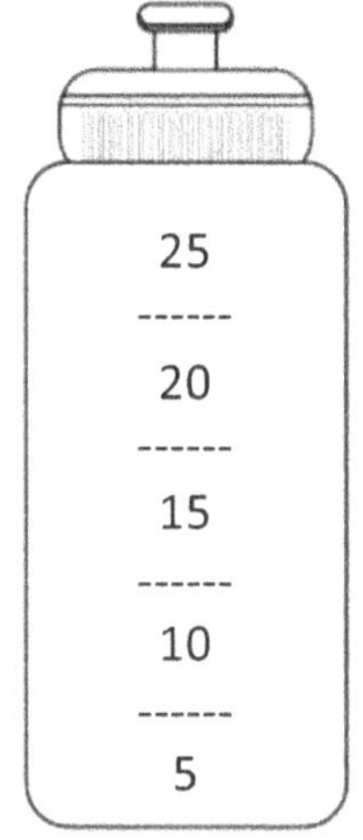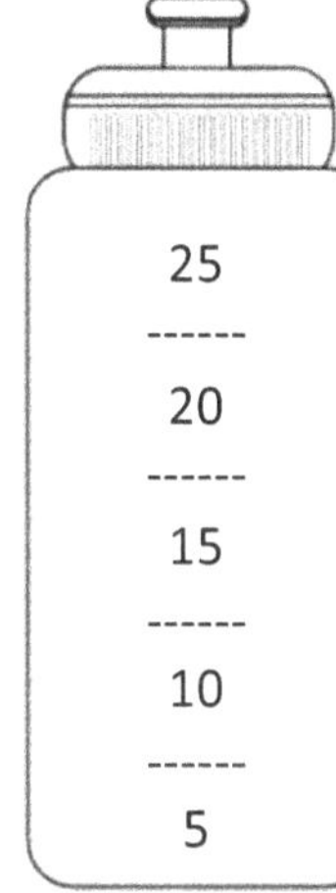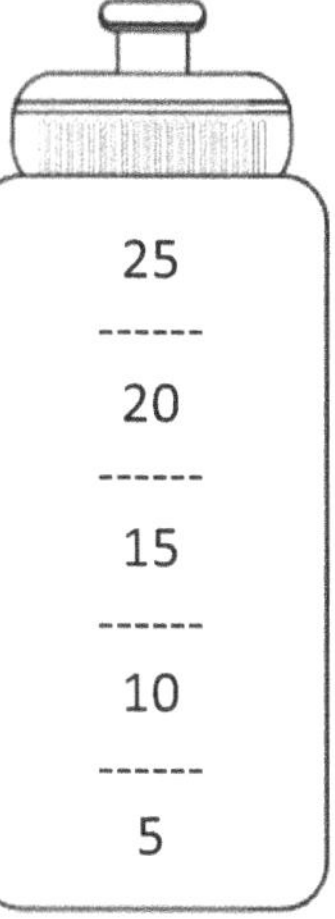

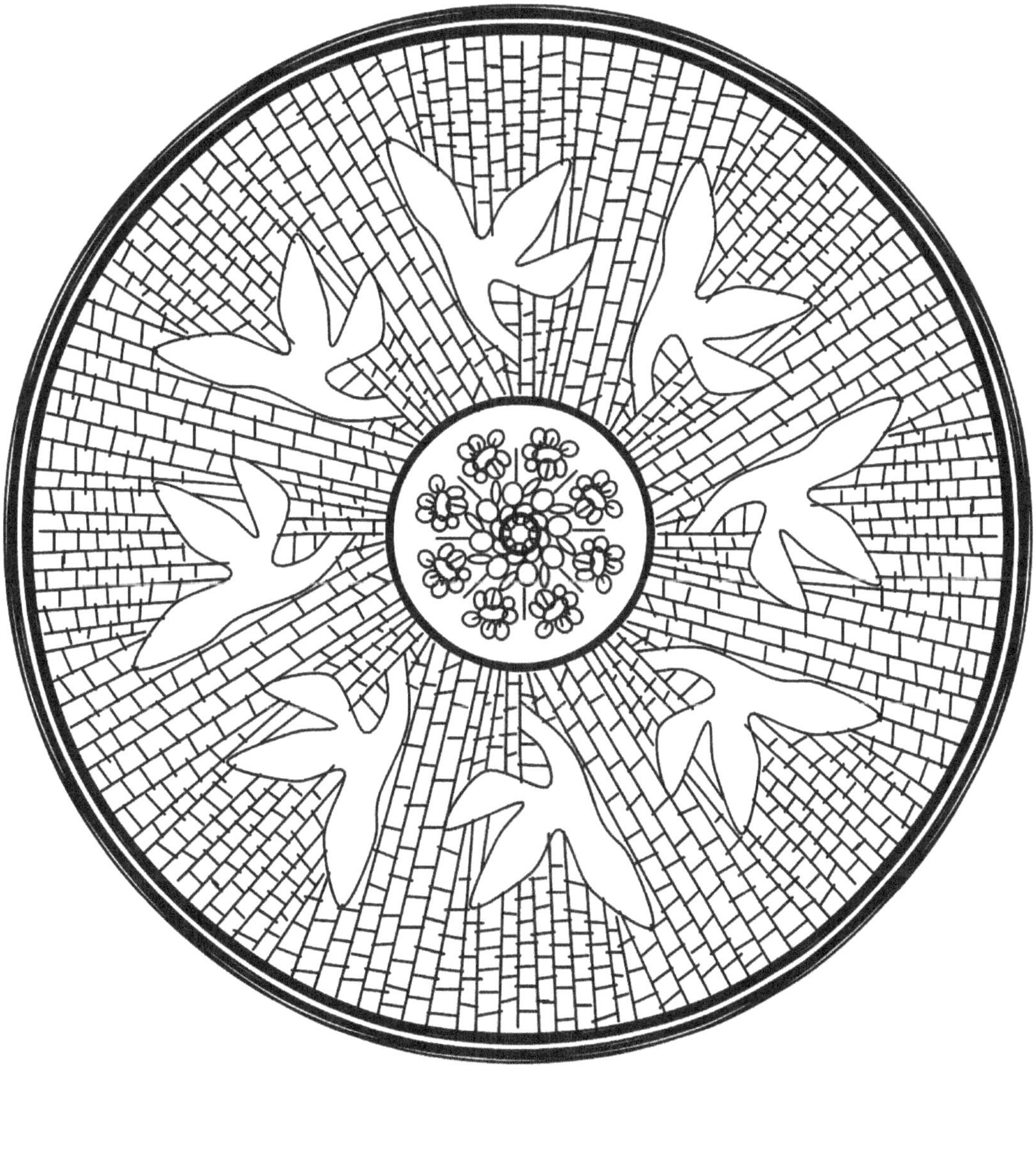

Measurements

DATE: ____________

Weight: _______

Neck _______

Shoulders _______

Chest _______

Bicep / upper arm left ________ right _______

Forearm left ________ right _______

Waist _______

Hips _______

Thighs left ________ right _______

Calf left ________ right _______

Only I Can Change My Life, No One Can Do It For Me!

Day Forty _______

5:00 _______________________

6:00 _______________________

7:00 _______________________

8:00 _______________________

9:00 _______________________

10:00 _______________________

11:00 _______________________

Noon _______________________

1:00 _______________________

2:00 _______________________

3:00 _______________________

4:00 _______________________

5:00 _______________________

6:00 _______________________

7:00 _______________________

8:00 _______________________

9:00 _______________________

10:00 _______________________

11:00 _______________________

Midnight _______________________

top priorities for today

____

____

____

____

Today's victories

Do you believe in magic or miracles?

____

____

____

____

____

____

The Stella Society Workout

Exercise	Set 1	Set 2	Set 3	Set 4	Set 5	notes

Time started: _____________ Time ended: _______________

Location: ____

Feelings before training:

Feelings after training

NUTRITION

Meal 1
time eaten: _________

Meal 2
time eaten: _________

Meal 3
time eaten: _________

Meal 4
time eaten: _________

Meal 5
time eaten: _________

Hydration

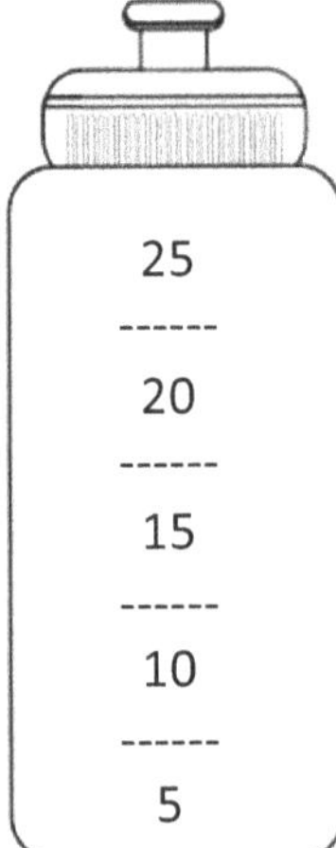
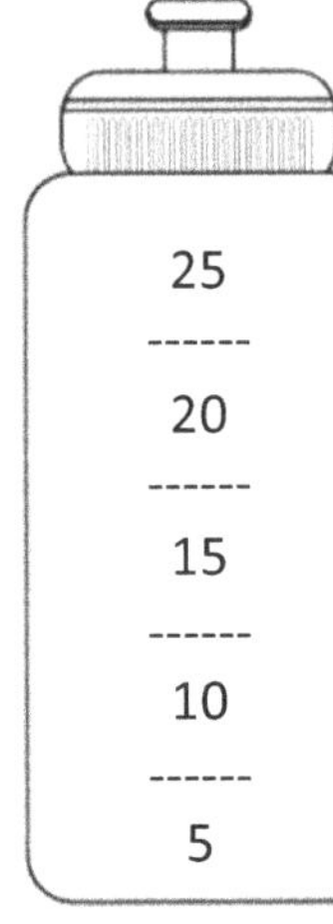
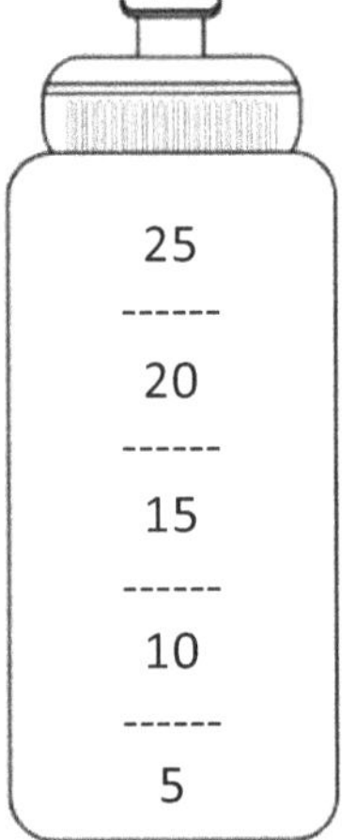
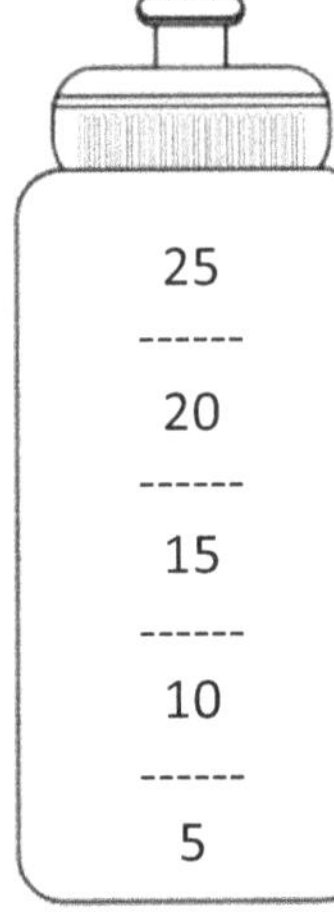
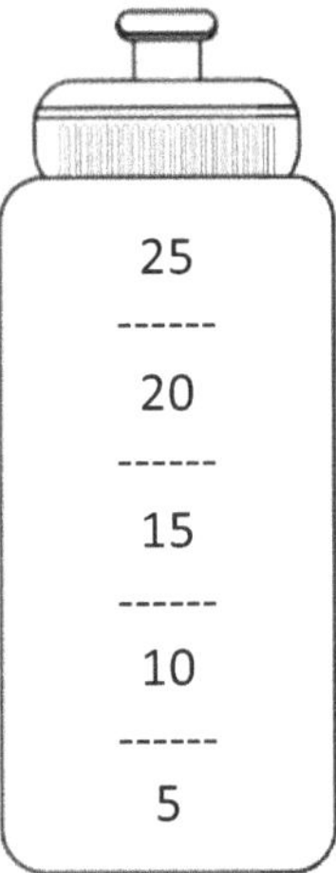

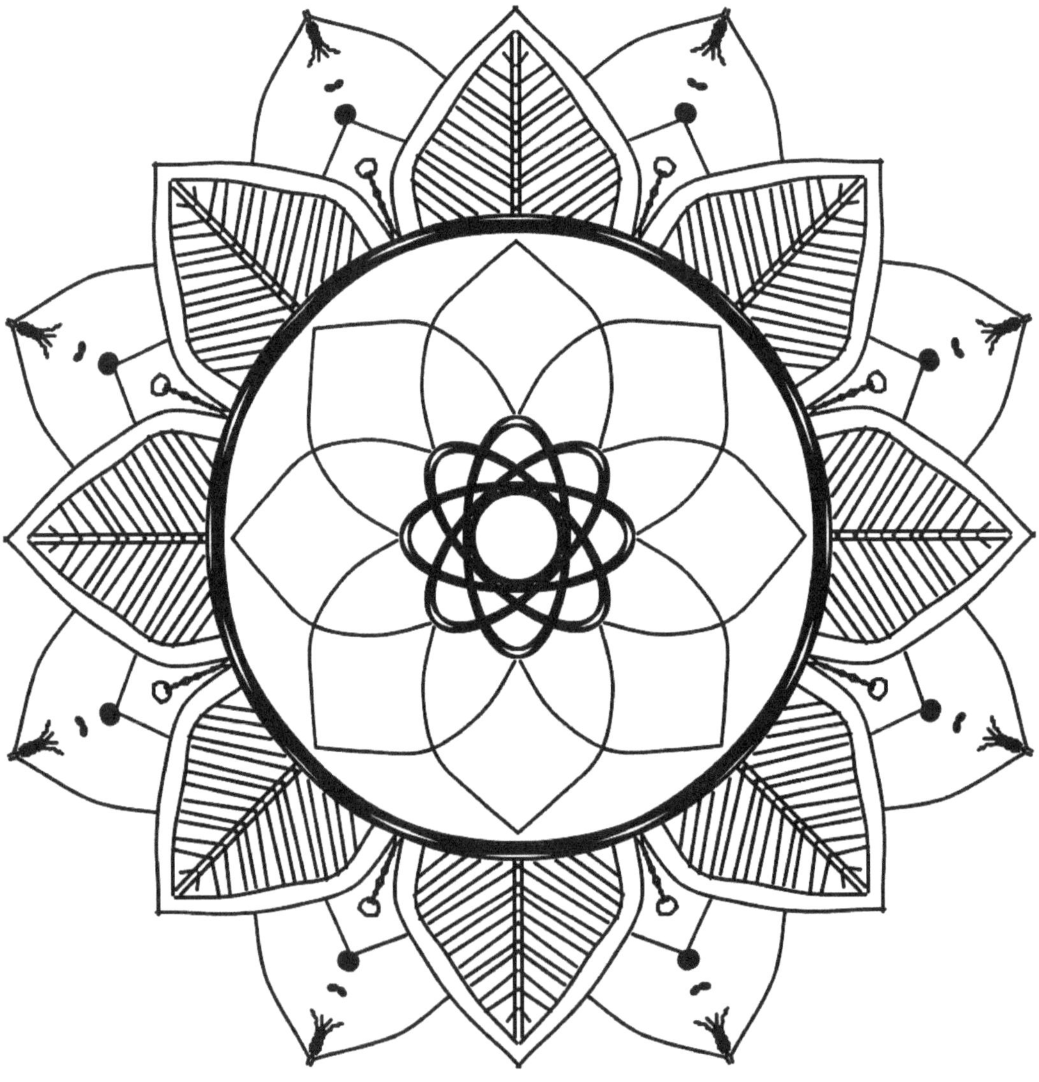

Day Forty-one ______

5:00 __________________________

6:00 __________________________

7:00 __________________________

8:00 __________________________

9:00 __________________________

10:00 _________________________

11:00 _________________________

Noon __________________________

1:00 __________________________

2:00 __________________________

3:00 __________________________

4:00 __________________________

5:00 __________________________

6:00 __________________________

7:00 __________________________

8:00 __________________________

9:00 __________________________

10:00 _________________________

11:00 _________________________

Midnight ______________________

Today's victories

What is one thing you want to do forever?

The Stella Society Workout

Exercise	Set 1	Set 2	Set 3	Set 4	Set 5	notes

Time started: ______________ Time ended: ______________

Location: ____

Feelings before training:

Feelings after training

NUTRITION

Meal 1

time eaten: _________

Meal 2

time eaten: _________

Meal 3

time eaten: _________

Meal 4

time eaten: _________

Meal 5

time eaten: _________

Hydration

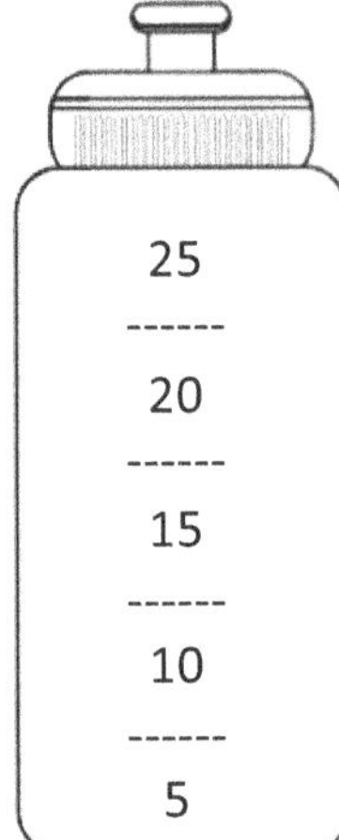

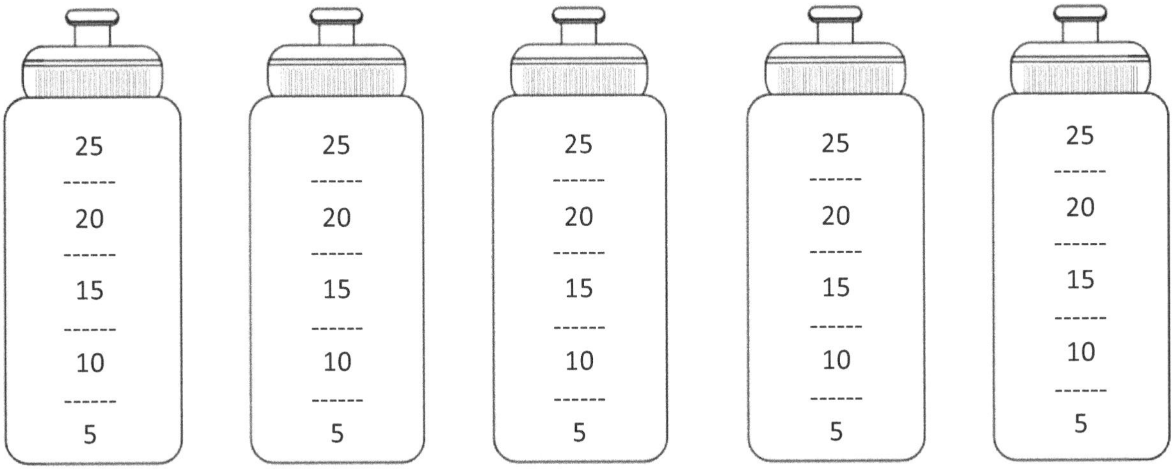

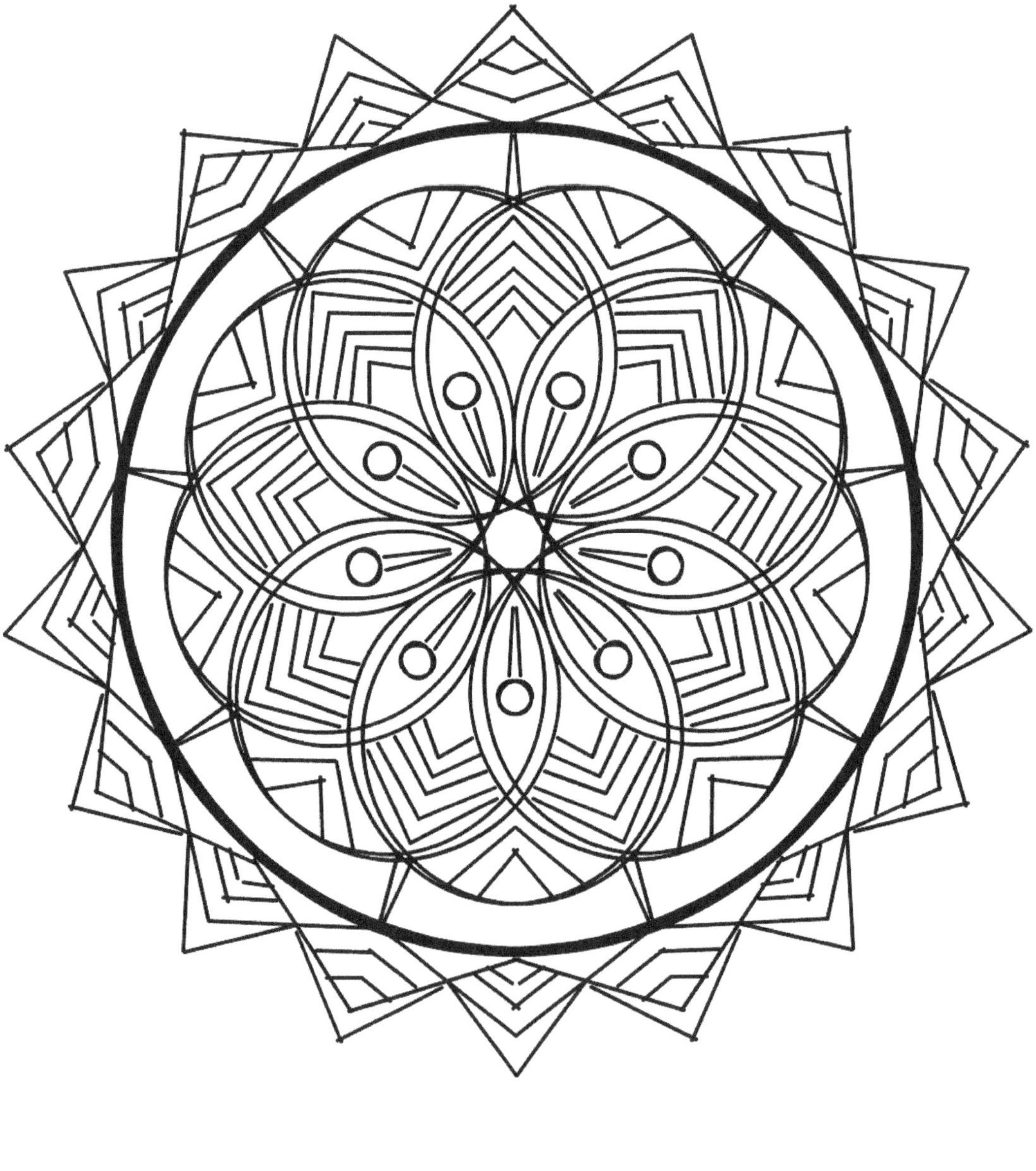

Day Forty-two _______

5:00 _______________________

6:00 _______________________

7:00 _______________________

8:00 _______________________

9:00 _______________________

10:00 _______________________

11:00 _______________________

Noon _______________________

1:00 _______________________

2:00 _______________________

3:00 _______________________

4:00 _______________________

5:00 _______________________

6:00 _______________________

7:00 _______________________

8:00 _______________________

9:00 _______________________

10:00 _______________________

11:00 _______________________

Midnight _______________________

top priorities for today

____

____

____

____

Today's victories

What was your biggest
victory in the last 40 days?

____

____

____

____

____

____

The Stella Society Workout

Exercise	Set 1	Set 2	Set 3	Set 4	Set 5	notes

Time started: _____________   Time ended: _______________

Location: ____

Feelings before training:

Feelings after training

NUTRITION

Meal 1

time eaten: _________

Meal 2

time eaten: _________

Meal 3

time eaten: _________

Meal 4

time eaten: _________

Meal 5

time eaten: _________

Hydration

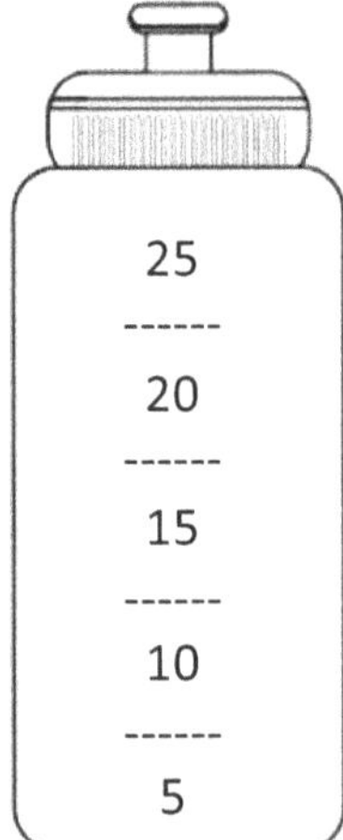

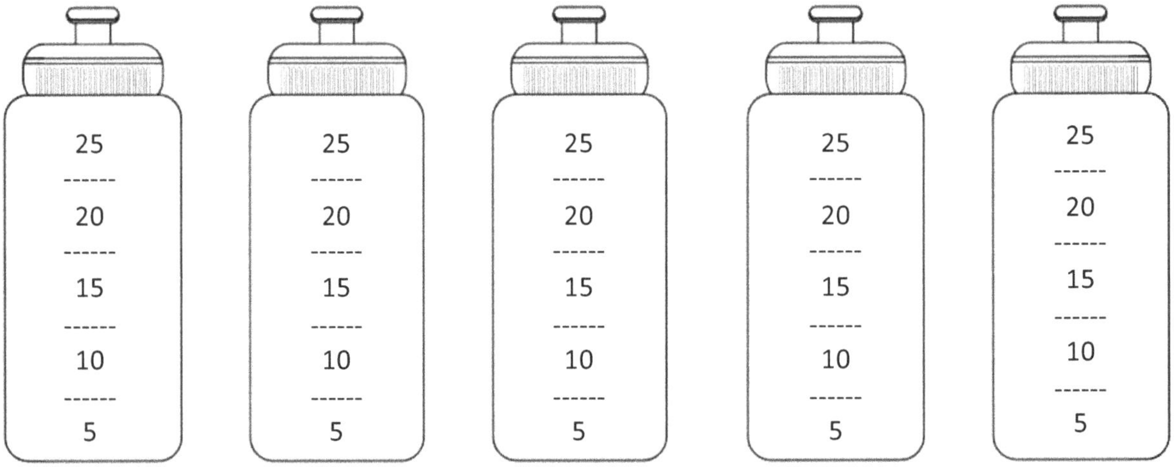

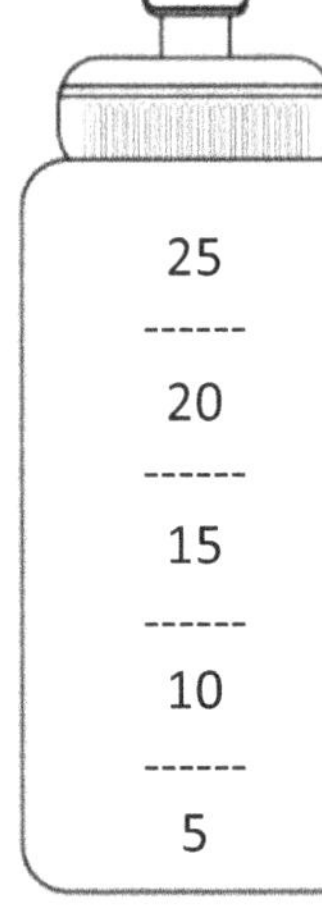

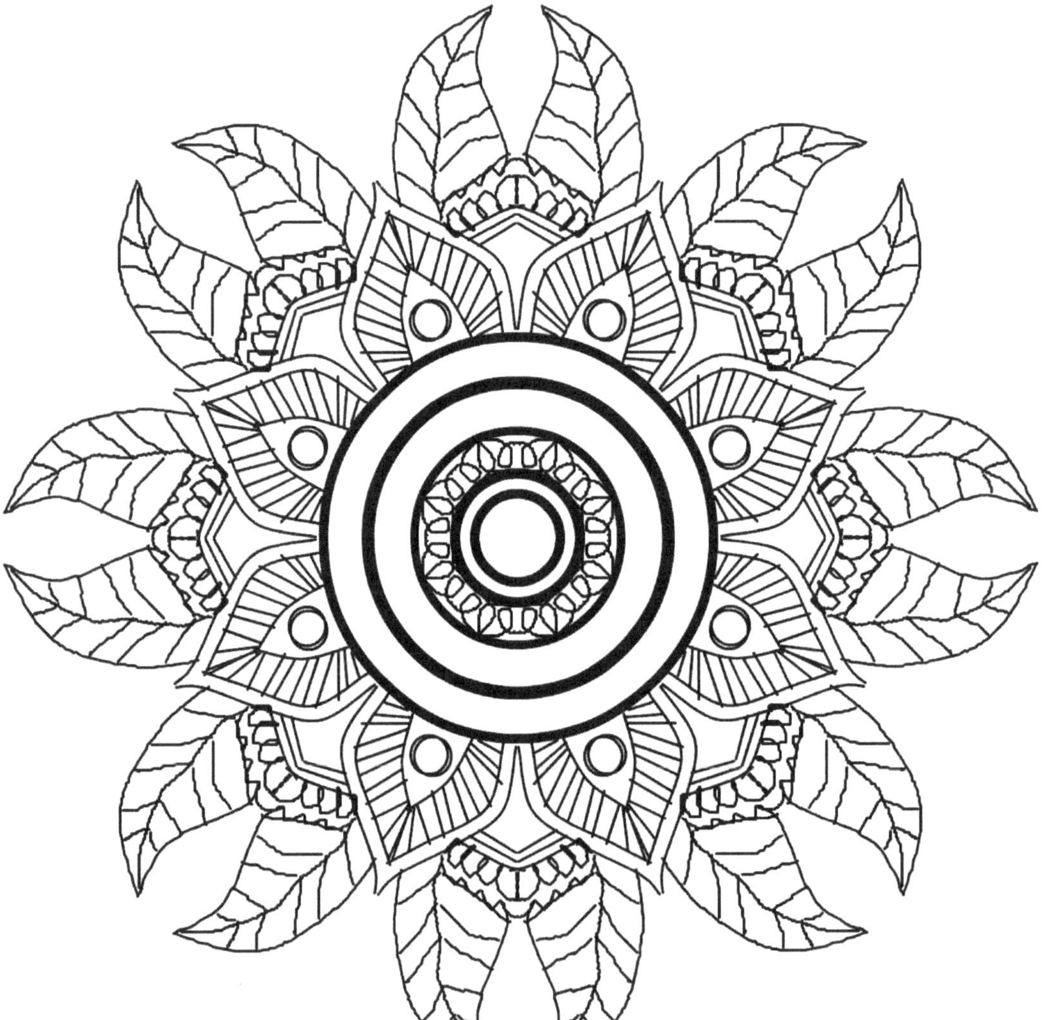

NOW WHAT?